BLACK

HEALTH

BLACK HEALTH:

CONSIDERED FROM A HOLISTIC PERSPECTIVE

D'Andrea M. Bolden, MA

Written Wisdom Press • Kalamazoo, Michigan

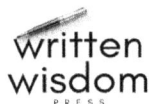

written
wisdom
PRESS

written
wisdom
PRESS

WRITTEN WISDOM PRESS
PO Box 2025
Kalamazoo, Mi 49003

Paperback ISBN: 979-8-218-03771-0
E-Book ISBN: 979-8-9881346-3-3

For more information about exclusive discounts for bulk purchases, please contact info@writtenwisdompress.com

Cover design by: Nfuxion Design Solutions

Cover illustration is protected by the 1976 United States

Copyright Act. Printed in the United States of America

Dedication

I want to dedicate this book to my parents, Mr. Ralph Cunningham, and Mrs. Bernice Cunningham. Without you there is no me. I want to thank you both for lending me your strong shoulders to stand on so that my feet never have to touch the ground. Love you always!

Thank you to my best friend and husband, John. Thank you for always pushing me every time I want to quit, which has been more frequent than I would like to admit... LOL

Thank you to my two wonderful children for making life a bit more colorful, and for causing me to live more wisely and with greater intention for the future. I pray that you are the arrows that hit the target.

Contents

Whole: Holistic Health

Other Health Concerns

Disclaimer

The full content of this book is limited to informational and entertainment purposes only. This is not in any way a replacement for professional medical or mental health advice, assessments, examinations, diagnoses, or treatment.

The reader (you) should consult a mental health or medical professional regularly in matters relating to your physiological health or mental health and particularly with symptoms that may require diagnosis or treatment.

Always seek the guidance of your doctor or other qualified health professionals with any questions you may have regarding your health or a medical condition. Never disregard the advice of a mental health or medical professional, or delay in seeking it because of something you read in this book.

If you think you may have a medical emergency, call your doctor, go to the nearest hospital emergency department, or call the emergency services immediately. If you choose to rely on any information provided in this book, you do so solely at your own risk.

Introduction
Purpose Of This Book

I have learned that health is wealth, and like many others I am now trying to rectify the years I spent not knowing this simple truth. Many people are unaware of how poor dietary and lifestyle choices can impact their physical health negatively. The same lack of knowledge can be applied to our mental health - especially when we are still fighting against stigmas and other misconceptions that keep people from seeking professional mental health services. Also, we need to learn the role that faith can play in our spiritual health and not misuse it to fix things that require professional care or some simple adjustments that we can make on our own.

As black people, our health is of great concern. In fact, many of our people lack trust in doctors and the healthcare system. We can all admit that this lack of trust was rightly earned as we reviewed closely many of the atrocities that occurred in the past. However, we see the need to share information that can help us evolve and transform so that we can safeguard our health as much as possible.

Health is a complicated topic for black people, with emphasis on all of us in the USA. The ugly truth and history of how black people were used as guinea pigs where they were brutally traumatized and tortured in the name of advancing science and medicine has left a bitter taste and a high level of skepticism in many. Those same individuals that were subjected to such abhorrent treatment were never able to experience the "benefits" that came from their blood, tears, and pain.

As we review the past, we can see the origin of the systems that are in place today, along with the mindsets that have perpetuated a disregard for black pain. From a historical lens we can also recognize the ever-present inequality and bias when it comes to accessing and receiving adequate, compassionate care. Sadly, those same attitudes and barriers are still alive today but have been repackaged and are now intellectualized and modernized. Consider how black pain is ignored as many working in healthcare are still in agreement with the lie that we do not feel pain in the same way as other groups of people.

The purpose of this book is to highlight some of the things that are having a significant impact on the health of black people overall, and to show accurate, up-to-date scientific information in a practical way so that anyone can understand. This book uses and references medical and scientific literature, but it is written for the average person and not exclusively those with advanced degrees or a background in healthcare and mental health.

I have attempted to write this in a way that is impactful but not intimidating to readers with pages filled with medical terminology and scientific language, which is not a good fit for the intended audience of this book. My main objective in authoring this book is to share understandable, relevant facts, and information in a simple manner.

I authored this book because I want to see more black people "woke" as far as their health, especially when there are some changes that many of us can make to protect our health, regardless of its current state. Unfortunately, sometimes we wait until things have gotten out of hand before we are willing to make changes.

Some can attest that over the years before health-related issues progressed, their doctors made suggestions for dietary changes and an increase in exercise, and it was all ignored. We must become more proactive and not just reactive.

Please note that I am fully aware that racial bias, healthcare disparities, and a lack of health equity all play a role in many of the health challenges that black people face. This is especially important for black women when you begin to consider maternal health, postpartum health, infant mortality rates, and maternal mortality rates. However, if you are reading this book, please know that I am not writing to focus solely or heavily on health disparities, health insurance and other barriers that we face as it pertains to quality care. Although those topics could not be avoided during the process of authoring this book, I want to focus more on things that we can learn, changes that we can make, and behaviors that we can break to see an upturn in black health overall because humans tend to value health only when illness is present.

As you are reading this book, you might notice that the terms black and African American are used interchangeably. I feel that the term "black" is more inclusive for those who are a part of the diaspora but are not living in America, or who are living in America but are not Americans by birth. However, this is written through the lens of the black American experience.

Although this book is written with a black audience in mind, I understand that the readership can include individuals that are not black. For this reason, I have included some things that are typically common knowledge within the black culture but could be unknown to non-black readers. So, keep that in mind as you read this book.

Lastly, there tends to be a lot of incorrect and confusing information on physical and mental health in the black community. Sadly, I have seen a lot of my black brothers and sisters believing lies while rejecting simple things that have been proven to be true. Over the past few years, the amount of bad information that I have seen my people falling for and embracing is heartbreaking. For instance, a few years ago I saw a discussion on an extremely popular social media platform where a group of adults were sharing how much aluminum foil to ingest to avoid issues caused by 5G. I was absolutely flabbergasted, and I could not believe that people would be duped so easily into believing that ingesting aluminum foil was helpful, not knowing the dangers that would cause to their health. Fear not; eventually, that terrible post was removed from the social media platform.

I have also seen a lot of charismatic people that have made false health-related claims to grow their online brands, knowing that some of their black audiences do not have a lot of accurate scientific knowledge that would help them to combat and dispute the false claims and the "snake oil" that they are trying to sell.

This book was not easy to write; but I tried my best, so here we go...

Do not make everything else a priority aside from your own health. Grinding and securing the bag will not matter much if your body and mind begin to "break down." – *D'Andrea Monet Bolden*

Body.

Physiological Health

This section of the book has multiple chapters that are relevant to the health of your physical body.

Chapter 1.
Common Issues We Face

The Office of Minority Health reported that the life expectancy is 79.8 for black women and 74.0 for black men. It was also shared that blacks die more often than whites do from strokes, HIV/AIDS, homicide, heart disease, pneumonia, influenza, cancer, and asthma.[1]

What are some of the most common health issues seen in the black population? Over the years it has been reported by the medical community that there are some health conditions that are seen often amongst the black population. We cannot and should not ignore these findings but instead we must become more open to learning about our family history, our individual health, and our bodies.

I am quite sure that anyone reading this book has heard of most, if not all, of the health conditions that I will mention in this chapter. However, I am not so sure that the same number of people understand the prevalence of these health conditions within the black population and how they can affect a person's quality of life and life expectancy. It is also important to know that these health disorders can increase the risk of developing or lead to other health issues when and if they continue to progress. I strongly believe that including all of them in this chapter will be beneficial to readers.

WHAT WE DO NOT KNOW CAN HURT US

I know that I am not the only one that was not raised in a health-conscious household. What I mean by this is that I grew up not being taught about nutrition, diet, exercise, and the need for regular doctor's visits. Many of us grew up in families where our ancestors were in survival mode, and they did the best that they could do. Now that we have more information and access to more resources, we can do better. Therefore, we can break the generational cycle of ignorance in our families by teaching the next generation about these things. The earlier we educate and incorporate these practices in our homes, the faster we can make improvements in our families and communities.

Many of us only went to the doctor as needed and we dreaded those appointments. The importance of health was and for some still is the furthest thing from our minds. Sadly, not all black people know the value or really consider the state of their health until it is too late. Many do not consider anything that they are putting in their body or their diet and lifestyle choices until they get shocking news from the doctor. Also, sometimes, even after getting a bad doctor's report, some individuals will remain unwilling to make any physician-mandated changes that could have a positive impact on their health.

It is no secret that African Americans still have a significant level of mistrust of doctors, hospitals, and anyone in a healthcare setting. Also, it is no secret that oftentimes we do not feel heard or feel that we are taken seriously and that the doctor has our best interest at heart. Health is wealth and it is invaluable, so it is necessary that we all select a health provider that is a good fit. This is not always easy, and you should not stop looking for a good fit until you are satisfied. There are a lot of great healthcare providers that will give you the compassionate care that you deserve. Knowing that you feel comfortable and have a positive experience with your healthcare provider makes a significant difference.

LEADING CAUSES OF DEATH

When I began authoring this book, I can admit that I was shocked by a lot of the information out there about the state of our health. However, I am glad that I have become aware and more educated about black health and the challenges that we are all facing.

The National Center for Health Statistics, and the National Vital Statistics System and Mortality shared the top five causes of death for black people (both genders, all ages) based on data from 2019 and they are listed below:

- Heart disease
- Cancer
- Accidents (unintentional injuries)
- Cerebrovascular diseases (e.g.: stroke, aneurysm)
- Diabetes

When we look at the top five causes of death of all ages separated by gender, the lists change a bit.

This is the top five leading causes of death for black males of all ages (2019):

- Heart disease
- Cancer
- Accidents (unintentional injuries)

- Cerebrovascular diseases (e.g.: stroke, aneurysm)
- Assault (homicide)

I thought it was worth sharing that the sixth leading cause of death for black males of all ages is diabetes.

Below are the top five leading causes of death for <u>black females</u> of all ages (2019):

- Heart disease
- Cancer
- Cerebrovascular diseases (e.g.: stroke, aneurysm)
- Diabetes
- Alzheimer's disease

For black females of all ages, the sixth leading cause of death is accidents (unintentional injuries).

COMMON HEALTH ISSUES WE FACE

Heart Disease

Heart disease is considered one of the leading causes of death - not just in the US but globally. The Center for Disease Control and Prevention (CDC) reported that about one in four deaths are attributed to heart disease annually.[2] The Office of Minority Health (OMH) reported that African Americans (AA) are thirty percent more likely than whites to die of heart disease.[3] So, what exactly is heart disease? Heart disease is a term that refers to a variety of heart-related conditions. Heart disease can be congenital (present at birth) or acquired during a person's lifespan.

Coronary artery disease, also referred to as coronary heart disease, is considered the most prevalent type of heart disease. Coronary artery disease is typically characterized by cholesterol deposits or plaque buildup in the arteries. Please note that arteries are blood vessels that carry blood towards your heart. Over time, these deposits can cause the arteries to become narrow which can limit blood flow to the heart.

There are several known factors that can increase the risk for heart disease[2]

- Diabetes
- High blood pressure (hypertension)
- High blood cholesterol
- Smoking
- Poor (unhealthy) diet
- Being overweight/obese
- Lack of physical activity/exercise
- Excessive use of alcohol

One thing I found very shocking was the prevalence of heart disease among African American women.[1-2] Did you know that an estimated 50,000 African American women die from heart disease annually?[2] Did you know that heart disease is the leading cause of death for African American women in the United States?[2-4]

One of the risk factors for heart disease is high blood pressure, and according to the Office of Minority Health, African American women are sixty percent more likely to have high blood pressure than white women.[2] They also shared African American adults are forty percent more likely than whites to have high blood pressure but they are less likely to have their blood pressure under control.[2] Research has not been able to explain fully why there are such differences with blood pressure when comparing non-Hispanic whites and non-Hispanic blacks.[4] There has been some evidence that supported the use of a sodium-restricted (low salt) diet to lower blood pressure in African Americans.[3]

The Office of Minority health shared that around 80% of African American women are overweight or obese and this is also a contributing factor to heart disease.[2] Now I know that everybody is not going to be a size two. I have not been that tiny since middle school; but as African American women, we can and should focus on being healthier by eating a better diet and becoming more active by walking and exercising on a regular basis.

High Blood Pressure

High blood pressure, which was listed as a contributing factor to heart disease, is one of the most common health issues and is seen in just over forty percent of African Americans over age eighteen. African Americans are also shown to develop high blood pressure that is more severe at a younger age when compared to other groups.[4] Some evidence backs the claim that some African Americans have a genetic component that makes them more sensitive to salt intake resulting in elevated blood pressure.[4] Higher rates of diabetes and obesity are also seen as possible causes for the high number of AA developing high blood pressure.

There are several risk factors for high blood pressure that should be mentioned. Family history (parents or other close blood relatives), age, gender, race (black), and chronic kidney disease are all factors that increase the chances of someone developing high blood pressure.

High blood pressure is considered a silent killer, and it can contribute to conditions that can lead to stroke and kidney failure. High blood pressure is so common that many do not take this diagnosis seriously. Many people are unaware that the progression of uncontrolled high blood pressure can increase the risk of heart attack, stroke, aneurysms, and atherosclerosis (thickening/hardening of arteries due to plaque buildup).

Cancer

I know the "c" word can be very upsetting and can be a trigger to people for a lot of reasons. I will make this section as short and informative as possible. Cancer is used to define several diseases that are characterized by the rapid out-of-control growth and spreading of abnormal cells.

When functioning properly, the body can destroy abnormal cells, but when cancer is present, the normal checks and balances within the body are not working as they normally should. Cancer in its various forms is something that affects people of all backgrounds around the world, but for whatever reason there are some significant statistics and valuable information about African Americans and cancer.

According to the American Cancer Society, blacks have the highest mortality rate and lowest survival rate for several types of cancers when compared to other ethnic/racial groups in the US, and black men have the highest cancer incidence rate.[5] There is no simple or single explanation for why these things have been found to be true. Socioeconomic factors, cultural factors, the quality level of accessible healthcare, and other factors are believed to play a role in the cancer rates seen among the black population.[5]

Cancer and black men

Top cancer sites for black men as listed by the Office of Minority Health, with the source being the National Cancer Institute,[6-7] are:

- Colon and Rectum
- Esophagus
- Kidney
- Liver and IBD (Intrahepatic Bile Duct)
- Lung

Individuals that are non-smokers and those who quit smoking lower their risk of lung cancer. Not smoking also reduces the chance of developing cardiovascular disease. It is important that black men have regular checkups and colonoscopies as suggested by a doctor to find any polyps or early signs of colorectal cancer.

Cancer and black women

Top cancer sites for black women as listed by the Office of Minority Health, with the source being the National Cancer Institute,[6-7] are:

- Breast
- Cervical
- Colon and Rectum
- Kidney
- Liver and IBD (Intrahepatic Bile Duct)

Typically, by the age of forty it is highly recommended that women begin scheduling mammograms. This can be especially important for the early detection of breast cancer. Breast cancer in African American women tends to develop at younger ages, have a poorer outcome and come in a more aggressive tumor type.[8] The mammogram screening rate for AA women is seventy-three percent and with early detection the mortality rate is reduced by almost fifty percent.[8] Hopefully more education and more awareness will help increase the rate of black women getting mammograms on a regular basis.

Type 2 Diabetes

I want to specify that this section is only referring to Type 2 diabetes. Diabetes is something that we have all heard of, and you might know someone that is diabetic. Type 2 diabetes is what happens when your blood glucose levels are consistently too high and the body either is not producing enough insulin or is insulin resistant. Insulin is what the body uses to help keep the blood glucose (sugar) levels from becoming too high which can lead to diabetes. When diabetes progresses, it can cause a lot of other health-related complications.

Signs of Type 2 Diabetes

- Fatigue
- Increased hunger and thirst
- Slow healing wounds
- Weight increase or decrease
- Vision problems
- Frequent urination

Diabetic complications can lead to several health challenges including heart disease, kidney disease, issues with the eyes, amputations, and nerve damage (neuropathy). I have personally witnessed several individuals be medically noncompliant with out-of-control blood sugar levels which caused many of the complications mentioned above. A lack of medical compliance includes not following the instructions of the physician. Things such as taking medication as prescribed and checking blood sugar levels as instructed are particularly important. While some adhere to taking medication, they might fall short on dietary changes and exercise mandates to yield the best results.

The risk for some of the complications associated with Type 2 diabetes can be reduced by adhering to the doctor's advice, going to regularly scheduled appointments and making the necessary dietary and lifestyle changes. Many of us are used to hearing that someone is diabetic, and it does not really seem important until things get out of hand. A lot of people have the mindset that medicine will do all the work with no other changes or actions necessary on their part.

The medical community believes that individuals with Type 2 diabetes can live a "normal" life as it is not considered a "death sentence." But as mentioned before, the complications associated with diabetes can impact a person's health and life expectancy. In some cases, adherence to doctor's advice and care can see blood sugar levels return to normally accepted values with the inclusion of proper diet and exercise.

Kidney Disease

Kidney disease occurs when the kidneys begin to lose their function. The kidneys act like a filtering system to make sure that waste and other things are removed from the body. When the kidneys are not working properly, toxins can build up in the body.

Chronic kidney disease is a serious condition that results in the loss of kidney function over time, and this can lead to kidney failure. Kidney failure is also known as end stage kidney disease. Kidney failure is when the kidneys cannot function well enough for an individual to survive without an organ transplant or dialysis.

Risk Factors and Causes

Kidney disease can have several probable causes and risk factors such as diabetes (number one cause of kidney failure), inflammation of the kidney, high blood pressure, kidney cysts, reoccurring kidney infections, genetic kidney diseases, and ingesting certain medications, such as NSAIDs (i.e. ibuprofen, naproxen etc.), long term.[9]

Other Risk Factors

- Being black
- Family history
- Overweight/obesity
- Age
- Cardiovascular disease
- Smoking
- Obstruction to the urinary tract

According to statistics, black people are nearly four times more likely than whites to end up with kidney disease, and black people make up thirty-five percent of all individuals in the US with kidney failure.[10] The increased risk of blacks developing kidney failure is partially attributed to the significant levels of diabetes and high blood pressure seen in the black population.[10] Hypertension (high blood pressure) was listed as the most common cause for the majority of blacks with renal failure.[11]

Kidney failure can require the introduction of renal replacement therapy such as dialysis. I have witnessed multiple family members and friends get to the point where dialysis was a necessity. Home-based dialysis and kidney transplantation are the top preferred renal replacement therapies but are less likely to be the treatments received by blacks.[13] The most common renal replacement therapy received by blacks is hemodialysis in a center.[12] With hemodialysis comes a few possible complications including anemia, muscle cramps, heart disease, diseases of the bone, high or low blood pressure, and water retention.

Without working kidneys, a person can only live for a brief period. The purpose of dialysis is to ensure that the excess waste and fluids that were not removed by the kidneys are removed from the body. Without properly functioning kidneys or dialysis, toxins will begin to build up to dangerous levels in the body which can lead to death if not treated.

Dialysis is considered a temporary solution with kidney transplantation being the goal for many. As I was working on this chapter, I read how over 100,000 individuals need an organ transplant, with the majority needing a kidney.[13] Also, sadly, a sizeable number of these individuals are black. This is not a shock since black people are more likely to have kidney failure than other groups. Although significant changes are supposed to be put in place, it is believed that black people are less likely to be put on transplant lists and even less likely to receive an organ transplant after being put on this list.[13]

Here are a few things I read about this topic. One is that people are more likely to find a match from someone with a similar racial background, and there is a significant need for more black organ donors.[13] The stated standard is that people are not matched by race and that there are many success stories of people with different races matching for a successful organ donation. However, it has been stated that having a large(r) pool of individuals of similar racial backgrounds increases the chance of finding a match.

**I do want to share that as of 2023 race is set to be removed from the calculation of the eGFR (glomerular filtration rate). It is believed this will help more black people have a better chance of receiving a transplant and to receive the proper diagnosis sooner. **

The fact that race was included when calculating eGFR for black people in the first place is appalling and another example of how we are still fighting bias everywhere.

Cerebrovascular Accident (CVA): Strokes

The US Office of Minority Health stated that blacks were fifty percent more likely to have a stroke when compared to whites.[14] They also shared that black men were seventy percent more likely to die of a stroke when compared to whites.[14]

A stroke is a cerebrovascular accident that is known to limit or reduce the blood supply to the brain. Limited or reduced blood supply also means that the brain will not receive enough oxygen and other nutrients, and this can lead to brain damage, as brain tissue can die. Strokes can occur when blood vessels become blocked (fatty deposits or blood clots) or when they burst or leak. Strokes can be classified as ischemic (caused by blockage), hemorrhagic (caused by bursting or leaking blood vessels), cryptogenic (unknown cause), and transient ischemic attack (temporary disruption, mini stroke).

Risk Factors for A Stroke

- Overweight/Obese
- Smoking
- High Cholesterol
- Hypertension (high blood pressure)
- Diabetes
- Cardiovascular Disease
- Substance Abuse (illicit drugs)
- Heavy Drinking
- Lack of Exercise
- Family History

Signs Of a Stroke

- Sudden numbness or weakness in the face, arms, or legs (typically on one side).
- Sudden slurred speech, difficulty speaking or understanding speech.
- Sudden problems with vision in one or both eyes

- Sudden difficulties with coordination, balance, walking, or dizziness.
- Sudden extremely severe headache with no apparent cause

If you or someone else exhibits potential signs of a stroke, it is important to get emergency medical care immediately. Every minute is crucial to limit any permanent damage related to lack of blood supply to the brain during a stroke.

A Note About COVID-19

I saw online where the Mayo Clinic listed COVID-19 as a risk factor for someone having a stroke. I was shocked, but it also made sense as there is research that sheds light on this scenario.[15] I recall listening to an audio conversation of medical professionals. Eventually, a black female doctor told her story about how COVID-19 was associated with her having a cryptogenic (unknown cause) stroke. When COVID-19 first took the world by storm they emphasized constantly that people with health conditions and compromised immune systems were most prone.

Many of us then saw the black community get hit hard, with our family and friends being diagnosed with COVID-19; and some even passed away. I never realized how much the lack of proper nutrition, exercise, poor diet, and other lifestyle factors has a lot of black people needing to work aggressively on improving their health. I pray that as black people we make the necessary lifestyle and dietary changes to improve and safeguard our health. I really hope that this chapter sheds light on some of the health challenges we are facing in the black community.

I am also hoping it has become a little clearer on how many symptoms and risk factors are associated with multiple health disorders and how health disorders can be associated with other health disorders.

Peripheral Artery Disease and High Cholesterol

Before I end this chapter, I want to mention two other health concerns that the black community should be aware of: peripheral artery disease (PAD) and high cholesterol.

PAD can occur when arteries that supply blood to the arms or legs (typically the legs) become narrow. Arteries become narrow due to fatty deposits in the arteries. This is also known as atherosclerosis. These fatty deposits can be a combination of cholesterol, fats, calcium deposits and other substances. The buildup of fatty deposits (plaque) can lead to a reduction of blood flow to the arms and legs. Severe untreated PAD can lead to blood flow blockage, intense pain, tissue loss (gangrene) or limb amputation.

Risk factors include diabetes, smoking, hypertension, high cholesterol, heart disease, stroke, atherosclerosis, and being over the age of sixty.

High Cholesterol

Cholesterol is naturally found in our cells and in general is not bad and serves a purpose in our body. Cholesterol plays a significant role within the cell membrane and is also used to help the body produce several substances including steroid hormones.[16] There are two main types of lipoproteins that help transport cholesterol throughout the body.

The first type is "good cholesterol," also known as high density lipoprotein (HDL) and the second is low density lipoprotein (LDL). HDL is considered "good" because it transports cholesterol to the liver where it is then broken down and eventually removed from the body. On the other hand, LDL transports cholesterol to the arteries where it can begin to build up. This buildup can increase the risk of atherosclerosis, heart attack, stroke, or peripheral arterial disease. Triglycerides is another term that you might have heard when referring to cholesterol. Triglycerides are a type of fat found in your blood, and when your triglyceride levels are high along with low HDL or high LDL this can also increase the risk of health concerns such as a heart attack.

Please know that this chapter is not an exhaustive list, but it highlights some of the more prevalent health issues impacting black Americans.

Chapter References

1. Office of minority health. Heart Disease and African Americans – The Office of Minority Health. https://minorityhealth.hhs.gov/omh/browse.aspx?lvl=4&lvlid=19.

2. Heart disease facts. Centers for Disease Control and Prevention. https://www.cdc.gov/heartdisease/facts.htm. Published September 8, 2020.

3. Lackland D. T. (2014). Racial differences in hypertension: implications for high blood pressure management. *The American journal of the medical sciences*, *348*(2), 135–138. https://doi.org/10.1097/MAJ.0000000000000308

4. American Heart Association. (2016, October 31). High blood pressure and African Americans. www.heart.org. Retrieved from

https://www.heart.org/en/health-topics/high-blood-pressure/why-high-blood-pressure-is-a-silent-killer/high-blood-pressure-and-african-americans.

5. American Cancer Society. *Cancer Facts & Figures for African Americans 2019-2021*.

6. NCI 2021. Seer Cancer Statistics Review, 1975-2018. Table 1.24 and SEER*Explorer

7. NCI 2021. Seer Cancer Statistics Review, 1975-2018. Table 1.25 and SEER*Explorer

8. Gathirua-Mwangi, W. G., Monahan, P. O., Stump, T., Rawl, S. M., Skinner, C. S., & Champion, V. L. (2016). Mammography Adherence in African-American Women: Results of a Randomized Controlled Trial. *Annals of behavioral medicine: a publication of the Society of Behavioral Medicine, 50*(1), 70–78. https://doi.org/10.1007/s12160-015-9733-0

9. Mayo Foundation for Medical Education and Research. (2021, August 19). *Hemodialysis*. Mayo Clinic. Retrieved from https://www.mayoclinic.org/tests-procedures/hemodialysis/about/pac-20384824

10. National Institute of Diabetes and Digestive and Kidney Diseases . Race, Ethnicity, & Kidney Disease.

11. Eggers P. W. (1995). Racial differences in access to kidney transplantation. *Health care financing review, 17*(2), 89–103.

12. Norris, K. C., Williams, S. F., Rhee, C. M., Nicholas, S. B., Kovesdy, C. P., Kalantar-Zadeh, K., & Ebony Boulware, L. (2017). Hemodialysis Disparities in African Americans: The Deeply Integrated Concept of Race in the Social Fabric of Our Society. *Seminars in dialysis, 30*(3), 213–223. https://doi.org/10.1111/sdi.12589

13. Jealous, B., Locke, J., & Segal, G. (2020, December 17). *New Organ Donation Rule Is A Win For Black Patients And Health Equity*. Health

Affairs. Retrieved from
https://www.healthaffairs.org/do/10.1377/hblog20201211.229975/
full/

14. *Office of Minority Health*. Stroke and African Americans – The Office
of Minority Health. (n.d.). Retrieved from
https://minorityhealth.hhs.gov/omh/browse.aspx?lvl=4&lvlid=28

15. Wijeratne T, Gillard Crewther S, Sales C, Karimi L. COVID-19
Pathophysiology Predicts That Ischemic Stroke Occurrence Is an
Expectation, Not an Exception-A Systematic Review. *Front Neurol.*
2021;11:607221. Published 2021 Jan 28.
Doi:10.3389/fneur.2020.607221

16. Zampelas A, Magriplis E. New Insights into Cholesterol Functions: A
Friend or an Enemy? Nutrients. 2019 Jul 18;11(7):1645. Doi:
10.3390/nu11071645. PMID: 31323871; PMCID: PMC6682969.

Chapter 2.

Does Stress Affect Your Health?

Can Stress Affect the Human Body?

Stress is important because anyone can relate to it regardless of personal differences. However, within the black community it is strongly believed that black people have a higher level of psychological distress.[1] This means that black men, women, and children are believed to be more stressed than non-blacks.

So, what exactly is stress? Stress can be defined as the body's response to an incident that causes emotional, physical, and psychological strain. Defining stress is important because stress can and will vary from person to person.

What is stressful to me might not bother someone else at all, and vice versa. Knowing what is stressful to you matters so that you can find ways to manage these things. We must learn how to cope with stress because life is full of situations and scenarios that can trigger a stress response in our body. A stress response refers to how the body reacts to something that is stressful to you. When the body is alerted to stress, the adrenal glands, which are located at the top of your kidneys, will release the hormones epinephrine (also referred to as adrenaline) and cortisol. When epinephrine and cortisol are released in the body, it can result in elevated blood pressure, increased heart rate and an increase of glucose in the blood. Although experiencing stress will happen, chronic stress is not good for the body, nor should it be seen as the norm.

According to Harvard Health, it is believed that chronic stress is associated with high blood pressure, elevated blood plasma sugar levels, anxiety, depression, addiction, obesity, and clogged arteries.[2] When I read this, I wondered how much of a role is stress playing in the overall health of black people. Black health is a tough topic to tackle as it is extremely complicated and there are so many layers to this, including the topic of stress.

Stress, like many other things, has a way of impacting the human body. Our bodies can handle stress, but our bodies are not made to deal with stress non-stop. Yet, many black people are dealing with chronic stress. Chronic stress is believed to be able to impact our nervous system and cause changes in the brain such as a decrease in brain weight and an atrophy of brain mass.[3]

Below are some common things that can be sources of stress in your life:

- Job – Your duties and responsibilities, including the number of hours you work and the time of day.
- Boss/Supervisor
- Finances/Bills
- Marriage/Your spouse
- Children
- Extended family (in-laws, siblings, cousins, etc.)
- Overextending yourself to others
- Racism
- Poverty (no running water, food scarcity, power shut off, housing instability)
- Neighborhood/Environment (gang activity, robberies, etc.)
- Trauma and abuse

Stress is a serious topic that should be addressed whenever discussing the topic of black health. One research study suggested that stress can be both a triggering and aggravating factor in disease.[3] This means that they believe that stress can be a factor in a person having an increased risk of onset or progression of disease.

Let us look at stress a little further. Stress can lead to the activation of the sympathetic nervous system (fight or flight sympathetic nervous system) and this is known to cause vasoconstriction which can lead to elevated blood pressure, blood clotting, and changes to blood vessels.[3] It is also believed that the immune system can be impacted by stress.[3] In very extreme cases some research has suggested that stress can be a factor in inhibiting the immune system to some degree which could allow the growth of cancer cells along with other notable changes associated with the development of cancer.[3-4]

Stress can come in multiple forms on the same day. Many of us have learned to live in survival mode. Black people have found multiple ways to keep going during adversity. I am proud of the resilience of our people, but the body and mind can only take so much.

Stress is associated with the release of a steroid hormone known as cortisol. The normal function of cortisol includes playing a role in immune function, the body's inflammatory response, stress response and metabolism.[5] However, chronic stress can be associated with gastrointestinal issues and a weakened immune system. Cortisol can raise blood pressure, increase blood sugar and the heart rate.[3] Although I knew stress was not good for you, I did not know that stress could affect your body in so many ways.

The black experience is one that is incredibly unique and sadly, it comes with its own set of stressors, and this includes racism in all its forms. Dealing with racism can be extremely frustrating and it can be a major source of stress by itself. This means that outside of life issues, socioeconomic status, family problems, and work, racism is another source of stress for black people.

I was excited and surprised to see multiple articles and studies addressing racism, mental health, and stress. However, I would like to see more research on the topic of racism as a source of stress and how it impacts the health of black people.

Chapter References

1. Lackland D. T. (2014). Racial differences in hypertension: implications for high blood pressure management. *The American journal of the medical sciences, 348*(2), 135–138. https://doi.org/10.1097/MAJ.0000000000000308

2. *Understanding the stress response*. Harvard Health. (2020, July 6). Retrieved from https://www.health.harvard.edu/staying-healthy/understanding-the-stress-response.

3. Yaribeygi, H., Panahi, Y., Sahraei, H., Johnston, T. P., & Sahebkar, A. (2017). The impact of stress on body function: A review. *EXCLI journal, 16*, 1057–1072. https://doi.org/10.17179/excli2017-480

4. Zhang L, Pan J, Chen W, Jiang J, Huang J. Chronic stress-induced immune dysregulation in cancer: implications for initiation, progression, metastasis, and treatment. Am J Cancer Res. 2020

May 1;10(5):1294-1307. PMID: 32509380; PMCID: PMC7269780.

5. Thau L, Gandhi J, Sharma S. Physiology, Cortisol. [Updated 2022 Aug 29]. In: StatPearls [Internet]. Treasure Island (FL): StatPearls Publishing; 2022 Jan-. Available from: https://www.ncbi.nlm.nih.gov/books/NBK538239/

Chapter 3.

What Are You Eating?

Does Your Diet Matter?

Who does not love good-tasting food? Tasty food makes you feel good, right? Like a lot of other black people, I grew up eating our beloved soul food. You know what I am talking about - fried pork chops, BBQ ribs, ham, macaroni and cheese (oven baked), yeast rolls, fried chicken, fried cabbage, collard greens, cornbread, cobbler, pound cake, sweet potato pie, and so many other dishes. Many of us would get super-excited in anticipation of the big Sunday dinners after church and during the holidays - because we cannot forget the feasts on the holidays.

I know that soul food makes us "feel good." It comforts us mentally, or maybe the anticipation of some delightful home cooking excites us. Since many of us ate the same diets, we should also notice how we saw some of the same health issues plague our individual families.

Traditional soul food is delicious, but is it good for your physical health? I emphasized traditional soul food because there are some new health-conscious and vegan variations of many of our delicious soul food dishes. But that is not what I am talking about; I am talking about the soul food that many of us grew up eating. Big mama would throw down in the kitchen all while having a litany of health issues. Some of those health issues could have been connected to diet. Fast food, processed foods, and foods that are loaded with sugar, butter and salt are not the best options if you want to be healthy. Excess carbs, piles of meat, and too much fat can work against our health. Now, diet alone is not necessarily the sole cause, but it could play a role in some health issues.

I can only speak for myself when I say that I have learned to get away from a lot of traditional soul food dishes and recipes. Do not get me wrong, I love good-tasting food like everyone else. However, I do not love it enough to continue eating that way, knowing that it could have negative implications on my health.

When you know better, you will do better. But is it that easy? I say no, it is not that easy to change the way you eat after eating a certain way for decades. After so many years you know what you want to eat, how you want it cooked, how it should be seasoned, and so on. Eating patterns, like many other patterns and habits in our life, are not easy to break. I am not one for restrictive diets and fads, especially when some of these well-advertised diets are frowned upon by the medical community and considered unsafe.

For the best advice on eating healthier, depending on the current state of your health, it would be wise for you to speak with your physician who can refer you to a nutritionist and dietitian. These are trained professionals that can help you learn how to eat healthier. Always talk to your doctor before engaging in any kind of extreme diet or making major dietary changes. This is important because you might have to limit or eliminate certain foods. The state of your health (diabetes, kidney disease, heart disease) can require some specific changes to what you eat regularly. In some cases, you could be required to adhere to a strict medical diet.

Now, some things are a no brainer. We all should know that your body does not need fast food and processed junk foods. I do not need to quote a scientific article to be confident in saying that junk food and fast food are enemies of your health. Excess fried foods, lots of sugar and high salt are also dietary no-no's for anyone. Although it is not considered food, avoiding excess consumption of alcohol is also important for one's health. Also, drinking water every day is important so that you stay properly hydrated.

I am not a dietitian by any means, but I wanted to share a list of foods that are considered healthier food choices. I have learned to never make assumptions about what other people know. So, I will not assume that people know what they should be eating. I have seen a lot of people grow up eating a diet of junk food and fast food every single day. So, to start making positive changes, some people might need some options of healthier foods that could be added to their diet.

Please note this is not an exhaustive list, instead these are just a few common food options.

FRUIT
Apples
Pomegranates
Blueberries
Bananas
Oranges
Watermelon

Grapefruit
Cantaloupe
Mangoes
Pineapples
Strawberries
Pears
Plums
Nectarines
Grapes
Cherries
Kiwi
Peaches
Honeydew Melon
Tomatoes

VEGETABLES + LEGUMES
Broccoli
Kale
Carrots
Spinach
Cabbage
Squash
Artichoke
Arugula
Asparagus
Cucumber
Pumpkin
Green Beans
Cauliflower
Navy Beans
quash
Greens (Collar, Turnip etc.)
Brussel Sprouts
Lentils

Peas
Chickpeas

WHOLE GRAINS
Whole Oats
Whole Wheat
Barley
Brown Rice
Quinoa
Bulgur

What we eat and what we drink is important. Staying hydrated and drinking water is something many people are not doing. A lot of adults how shared with me that they never drink water. I think more people to understand that drinking water should not be an option but something that is done consistently on a regular basis.

The Benefits of Drinking Water

Drinking water is so important to keep our bodies hydrated. Personally, I did not start drinking water until I was an adult in my 20s, but now it is what I drink most of the time. Aside from water I will drink tea, and on occasion I will drink a cup of coffee, and even less often will I have a sip of juice or lemonade, but that is rare. Ironically, there are still a lot of adults that do not want to drink water, instead they prefer carbonated beverages and other sugary drinks.

I can admit that I used to drink soda every single day but eventually I stopped. The more I learned about the benefits of drinking water, the more I made it a personal requirement to drink more water.

Drinking water:

- Helps your body with temperature regulation
- Helps with waste removal
- Keeps joints lubricated; cartilage found in joints are 80% water[1]
- Is important for the kidneys
- Helps the digestive system; dehydration can lead to constipation
- Helps to manage blood pressure
- Helps to cushion sensitive tissues as well as the brain and spinal cord
- Blood is fifty-five percent plasma, and ninety percent of blood plasma is water.[2]

Iron

I can remember hearing as a little girl that you need to take your daily vitamins. It did not seem important until I learned the significant role that vitamins and minerals can play in our body.

For instance, we all know someone that sits and chews ice religiously. Some people even have their own ice machines. I remember when I was pregnant with my son, I had to have ice all day, every day. What I eventually discovered is that some of the people that crave and eat ice (pagophagia) have low iron levels and this can occur with or without being anemic. Iron is a mineral that plays a key role in our lives.

Anemia is a condition noted for a lack of red blood cells and it can be caused due to low iron levels. But did you know that iron is used to make hemoglobin, which is a protein in red blood cells that helps to transport oxygen to your body? Both black men and women suffer from anemia more than other groups. Also, there is research that suggests black men and women have lower levels of hemoglobin.

Anemia should not be ignored because it can be associated with several health conditions such as cancer or kidney disease. Also, anemia can increase the risk of heart and lung health complications. With so many black women already at risk for heart disease, it is important to ensure that iron levels are adequate.

Foods that are considered a source of iron:

- Red meat
- Seafood
- Beans and lentils
- Spinach
- Nuts and seeds
- Green peas

VITAMINS AND MINERALS: NECESSARY SUPPLEMENTS

Minerals

Minerals are inorganic substances that are found naturally in the earth and in foods. Ingesting minerals is important to ensure that your body is healthy and functioning properly. Minerals play a role in many aspects of your body, including your immune system[3] and the contraction of your muscles.

Below is a list of some of the minerals that your body uses on a regular basis:

Calcium, phosphorus, potassium, sodium, chloride, magnesium, iron, zinc, iodine, chromium, copper, fluoride, molybdenum, manganese, and selenium.

Unlike minerals, vitamins are organic substances that are found in several edible sources such as fruits, vegetables, and beans. Many vitamins have a role in enzyme-catalyzing reactions in the body. Vitamins metabolize carbohydrates and proteins, and they can be involved with cell reproduction (and growth).

Below is a list of _some_ of the important vitamins that your body uses and needs on a regular basis:

Vitamins A, C, D, E, K, and the B vitamins (thiamine, riboflavin, niacin, pantothenic acid, biotin, B_6, B_{12}, and folate)

Other Supplements

- Omega-3 is a polyunsaturated fat which is considered a good/healthy fat; it has been reported as highly beneficial for heart health and inflammation reduction. Omega-3 (fatty acid) is another important supplement that can be found in fish, nuts/seeds, fish oil and in some foods that have Omega-3 added. This is not produced in the body and must be introduced by food and supplements. There are three types of Omega-3 fatty acids:

1. **EPA (eicosapentaenoic acid).** EPA is found in fish.*
2. **DHA (docosahexaenoic acid).** DHA is found in fish.*
3. **ALA (alpha-linolenic acid).** ALA is found in plants.*

*Several people like me are allergic and cannot consume fish to get the Omega-3 benefits. Be sure to talk with your doctor before taking any supplement.

- Turmeric is derived from a plant (Curcuma longa) and is promoted as being beneficial for skin, the digestive system and for having anti-inflammatory effects.

Always speak with your doctor before taking any kind of supplement to ensure that there is no interference with medications or potential side effects. Also, your doctor can let you know if what you are taking is valuable to your health as they are aware of the current state of your health.

Gut Health

Gut health is comprised of your digestive system along with the microorganisms of your gut. Over the years there has been a significant increase in research that emphasizes the importance of gut health and how it affects your health.

Research suggests that gut health can have an impact on the overall physical health of individuals. Researchers have also shared that our diet, or the food we eat, can have an impact on the bacteria (microbiota) in our gut.[4] It is important that bacteria in your body are balanced (good and bad bacteria). An excess of bad bacteria (i.e., Staphylococcus, and Escherichia coli) can throw things off balance. When the bacteria of the gut are balanced correctly there will be more healthy bacteria than bad. However, when the bad bacteria outnumber the good, it can result in several issues in the body.

It is believed (supported by science) that poor gut health can be associated with the development of gastrointestinal issues, Type 2 diabetes, and cardiovascular disease.[5-6] The promotion of prebiotics and probiotics has become more common; in fact, my own PCP suggests that her patients take probiotics.

I never realized how important gut health is to your total health. I am learning more about how our diet plays a huge role in our gut health. There is no excuse; we can no longer avoid cleaning up our diet. My suggestion is that we all make the necessary changes sooner than later.

Chapter References

1. Sophia Fox, A. J., Bedi, A., & Rodeo, S. A. (2009). The basic science of articular cartilage: structure, composition, and function. *Sports health*, *1*(6), 461–468. https://doi.org/10.1177/1941738109350438

2. InformedHealth.org [Internet]. Cologne, Germany: Institute for Quality and Efficiency in Health Care (IQWiG); 2006-. What does blood do? [Updated 2019 Aug 29]. Available from: https://www.ncbi.nlm.nih.gov/books/NBK279392/

3. Weyh C, Krüger K, Peeling P, Castell L. The Role of Minerals in the Optimal Functioning of the Immune System. Nutrients. 2022 Feb 2;14(3):644. doi: 10.3390/nu14030644. PMID: 35277003; PMCID: PMC8840645.

4. Zhang YJ, Li S, Gan RY, Zhou T, Xu DP, Li HB. Impacts of gut bacteria on human health and diseases. Int J Mol Sci. 2015 Apr 2;16(4):7493-519. doi: 10.3390/ijms16047493. PMID: 25849657; PMCID: PMC4425030.

5. Li WZ, Stirling K, Yang JJ, Zhang L. Gut microbiota and diabetes: From correlation to causality and mechanism. World J Diabetes. 2020 Jul 15;11(7):293-308. doi: 10.4239/wjd.v11.i7.293. PMID: 32843932; PMCID: PMC7415231.

6. Tang WH, Kitai T, Hazen SL. Gut Microbiota in Cardiovascular Health and Disease. Circ Res. 2017 Mar 31;120(7):1183-1196. doi: 10.1161/CIRCRESAHA.117.309715. PMID: 28360349; PMCID: PMC5390330.

Chapter 4.
Why Does Exercise Matter?

Physical activity or exercise is especially important for health, but not everyone understands that this can be the key to safeguarding your health. We hear about diet and exercise all the time but putting it into action is not always easy. It takes discipline to eat healthier on a regular basis and to exercise. Discipline is necessary because that is all that you will have once your motivation is low.

Living a sedentary life for a lot of people just happens. No one wakes up one day and decides to be a lazy person – at least, I hope that no one does that. What happens with most of us is once you get out of school, you get an adult job, and then you are grinding non-stop in this rat race, trying to get ahead in life.

As you get older you might begin to gain weight, especially women after bearing children. You look in the mirror and glance at old pictures, and you think, *where did all this weight come from over the years?* Also, for some of us you then think, *let me try and get this weight off by hitting the gym and working out.*

I have lost count of the adults that say the slogan, "New year, new me." At the start of a new year, they get a gym membership, and they go strong for one month or so, and then it is back to the old sedentary lifestyle for one reason or another. It could be lack of motivation, stress, or just feeling too tired to go.

For years I found myself in the cycle of starting and stopping exercise until I decided that exercising was necessary and that it was no longer an option. Exercise alone saves lives because it is not only good for our physical health, but also our mental health. Exercising and trying to work on your physical health is not easy. This could be one reason people give up or try to find shortcuts. However, finding a way to get motivated and disciplined enough to exercise on a regular basis will be beneficial especially as you get older.

It took hiring a personal trainer for me to become consistent. Now I know that someone might be thinking that they cannot afford to hire a trainer. There are several solutions - such as working out at home using free online videos on social media platforms (Facebook, YouTube, fitness apps, etc.). Currently, you can find a variety of online trainers that livestream their workouts for free. Another option is working out with a group of friends or taking a free fitness class. If you have a group of friends, you could find a trainer that you can pay hourly and split the cost. If none of these options work, try and find an accountability partner or give yourself a goal and a deadline to try and stay on track.

Types of Exercise

1. Stretching/Flexibility – Exercises to increase flexibility, mobility, and range of motion.
2. Strength – Exercises to improve strength and endurance
3. Aerobic/Cardio – Exercises that help with stamina and are great for cardiovascular health. It is believed that cardio exercises can help individuals have a lower resting heart rate. This can mean that your heart does not have to work so hard.
4. Balance – Exercises that are good for your balance by focusing on your legs and your core.

According to the CDC, National Institute on Aging, the Mayo Clinic, and Medical News Today, being physically active is beneficial for[1-4]:

- Brain health
- Weight management
- Lowering your risk for disease or combatting health conditions such as:
    - Cardiovascular disease
    - Type 2 diabetes
    - Stroke
    - Depression
    - Anxiety
    - Some forms of cancer
- Increasing the strength of your bones and muscles
- Boosting your energy
- Improving your daily activity
- Improving your mood
- Helping with sleep
- Improving your sexual health
- Increases your chances of living longer

I know that I am not the only person that knew exercise was good for your health and remained a lazy person. However, I decided that being active was a requirement for my life and that it was no longer an option. When you are working, raising kids, and super-busy on a regular basis, it can be hard to find time and energy to exercise. But once I implemented time management practices and started getting my life more organized, finding time to exercise was easy. And I know it is hard to believe, but once you start exercising on a regular basis, you will feel more energized. Getting started is the hardest part, but with exercise having so many benefits, putting it off is no longer an option.

Since the start of this book, I have lost thirty pounds and now I exercise on a more consistent basis. I began to understand that getting healthier requires a mind change, and your diet and lifestyle changes will follow.

With exercise it is easy to get discouraged, but just try and do something consistently. You can start off by walking every day, jumping rope, or riding an exercise bike. Whatever you choose, you can start small and be consistent. Over time you can increase the length and level of difficulty of your exercise routine.

Chapter References

1. U.S. Department of Health and Human Services. (n.d.). *Real-life benefits of exercise and physical activity*. National Institute on Aging. https://www.nia.nih.gov/health/real-life-benefits-exercise-and-physical-activity

2. Daniels, L. (n.d.). *The benefits of exercise for your physical and mental health*. Medical News Today. Retrieved January 15, 2023, from https://www.medicalnewstoday.com/articles/benefits-of-exercise

3. Mayo Foundation for Medical Education and Research. (2021, October 8). *7 great reasons why exercise matters*. Mayo Clinic. Retrieved January 15, 2023, from https://www.mayoclinic.org/healthy-lifestyle/fitness/in-depth/exercise/art-2004838

4. Centers for Disease Control and Prevention. (2022, June 16). *Benefits of physical activity*. Centers for Disease Control and Prevention. https://www.cdc.gov/physicalactivity/basics/pa-health/index.htm

Chapter 5.

Is Sleep Important For Your Health?

I am done with the "lose sleep and grind it out" culture. It is not for me because I choose my health, peace, and happiness over losing sleep to reach a bar that is getting higher. I will not ignore my body's signals that I am tired, and there is no need to grind all day, every day. I do not judge or knock anyone who feels the need to grind and sleep less; that is their right. It is not for me, and it is not something that I will promote.

I know that I am not the only one that has heard people say that to be successful you need to forego a good night's rest. Well, I used to agree with that way of thinking, but what good is "success" if it will cost you your health? Rest is not an option; it is necessary, and your body needs to get a good amount of rest. By now you should recognize that your body gets tired for a reason, and that there are health benefits in getting enough sleep.

I have always heard that getting an adequate amount of sleep is important, but I was never really told any of the benefits of sleep. Did you know that getting enough sleep is important for your body to keep steady blood sugar levels? If you knew this already, then good for you because I was certainly unaware of sleep having a positive impact on blood sugar levels. In fact, it is believed that getting enough sleep can help reduce your chances of developing Type 2 diabetes.[1] Obviously there are still other factors involved in the development of Type 2 diabetes, but getting enough sleep does not work against you.

Also, getting enough sleep can be beneficial for the maintenance of your weight. This is because getting enough sleep is believed to make you feel less hungry.[1] According to the CDC, a lack of sleep can increase the risk for high blood pressure and heart disease. [2] Currently it is suggested that adults get at least seven hours of sleep per day. Unlike adults, children and teens need more hours of sleep per day, with the suggested amount between nine and twelve hours for ages six to twelve, and eight to ten hours for teenagers.[3]

I had to readjust my thinking and start making sleep a priority. You can lack mental sharpness without adequate sleep. Did you ever notice that when you get tired you tend to make more mistakes? A lack of sleep can throw off your mood. If you go without sleep long enough, you can become irritable and quite grumpy.

If you struggle to fall asleep, stay asleep, or you always feel tired, be sure to reach out to your healthcare provider. Some issues with sleep could be caused by a condition that requires evaluation, diagnosis, and treatment by a professional.

Also, for those that struggle to fall asleep, there are several apps and video channels that make music and videos to help you fall and stay asleep. I have tried apps and video channel options, and they worked fine.

Chapter References

1. Ellis, R. R. (2021, June 12). *7 surprising health benefits to getting more sleep*. WebMD. Retrieved January 19, 2022, from https://www.webmd.com/sleep-disorders/benefits-sleep-more

2. Centers for Disease Control and Prevention. (2021, January 4). *How does sleep affect your heart health?* Centers for Disease Control and Prevention. Retrieved January 19, 2022, from https://www.cdc.gov/bloodpressure/sleep.htm

3. Centers for Disease Control and Prevention. (2020, September 10). *Sleep in Middle and high school students*. Centers for Disease Control and Prevention.

Chapter 6.
Do Health Checkups Matter?

How often do you go to the doctor? When was the last time you had blood work done? Did you visit the doctor regularly as a child? Do you have a primary care provider? Why do health checkups matter? Why is disease prevention important?

Preventative care in the form of health checkups and screenings help with early detection and catching potential health issues before they develop into something serious. Regular doctor visits and screenings can allow health conditions to be discovered in the initial stages before they progress. Preventative care includes measures taken for the prevention of disease, death, and disability.

Examples of Preventative Healthcare

- Education on topics such as weight loss and smoking cessation
- Mammograms, colonoscopies
- Regular well child visits
- Screening for cancer or diabetes
- Cholesterol tests
- Mental health evaluations
- Tests for sexually transmitted illnesses
- Checking blood pressure

Some preventative healthcare screenings are typically recommended after a certain age or after a certain amount of time has passed since the last check.

I know that visiting the doctor for some people can put them in a bad mood or they can become extremely nervous for a lot of reasons. Some people may avoid regular doctor's visits to ensure that they do not receive any unwelcome news. I have seen this happen, especially when individuals were having some serious symptoms such as the inability to produce a bowel movement for weeks at a time or lots of bright red blood in their stool. I know that things can be very scary at times, but we cannot ignore our bodies, especially when going to the doctor could save our lives.

There are several studies and articles that address the topic of black preventative care. In fact, results in the past have been mixed when comparing the rates of blacks and whites that receive preventative care.[1] Socioeconomic status (SES) was shown to complicate matters when considering racial disparities and preventative care. One thing they shared is that because a considerable number of black men are considered to have a lower SES, this plays a role in the preventative care results, and along with race, this makes it difficult to discern how they affect preventative care rates individually. Those with a lower SES are believed to seek healthcare less often except for emergencies.

Being black has its own set of challenges as it pertains to healthcare. In addition, earning a low income has its own set of challenges. A lot of low-income individuals either have Medicaid, Medicare, or are completely uninsured. This can play a role in access to healthcare services and how often people seek out services. Tens of millions of American adults do not have health insurance or are inadequately insured.

Although preventative care can lower the chances of death, disease, and other health complications, it is believed that millions of people do not receive preventative care.

The Office of Disease Prevention and Health Promotion has listed several preventative care objectives that they are striving to achieve by 2030. Examples of these objectives include increasing the number of children that undergo developmental screening, and increasing the total number of community-based organizations that offer preventative care services.

The goal should be for more black and low-income individuals to get screened regularly to identify potential health concerns before they progress. This could lower the statistics regarding black people and certain healthcare issues.

Chapter References

1. Thorpe, R. J., Jr, Bowie, J. V., Wilson-Frederick, S. M., Coa, K. I., & Laveist, T. A. (2013). Association between race, place, and preventive health screenings among men: findings from the exploring health disparities in integrated communities study. *American journal of men's health*, *7*(3), 220–227. https://doi.org/10.1177/1557988312466910

2. Becker, G., & Newsom, E. (2003). Socioeconomic status and dissatisfaction with health care among chronically ill African Americans. *American journal of public health*, *93*(5), 742–748. https://doi.org/10.2105/ajph.93.5.742

"We have the tendency to value health once illness comes along. Let us be proactive and not just reactive." – **D'Andrea Monet Bolden**

Soul.

Mental Health

This section of the book is about your (soul) mental health: emotional and psychological wellbeing.

Chapter 7.
What Is Mental Health?

Mental Health Definition: According to the World Health Organization (WHO), "mental health is a state of mental well-being that enables people to cope with the stresses of life, realize their abilities, learn well and work well, and contribute to their community."

The terms mental health and mental illness (now known as mental health disorders) are oftentimes used interchangeably, but they are not the same.

Mental Illness Definition: Mental illness (mental health disorders) refers to a variety of *mental* disorders that affect your mood, thinking and behavior[+]

   [+]The term mental illness is being used less and is being replaced by mental health disorder.

Mental illness can be very debilitating and can interfere with an individual's ability to function from day to day and do things such as work, care for small children, and maintain stable housing and employment.

Mental health has everything to do with our emotional and psychological well-being. According to the National Alliance on Mental Illness, one in five adults in the US will be diagnosed with a mental health disorder annually. However, addressing your mental health does not mean that you will meet the criteria automatically to be diagnosed clinically with a mental health disorder.

Mental health disorders can affect a person's mood, thinking, and behavior over time. These disorders are diagnosed and treated by state-credentialed mental health professionals with the aid of the Diagnostic and Statistical Manual of Mental Disorders (DSM-V) fifth edition, and other tools. The DSM-V is used by professionals as it contains the classification of current mental health disorders along with the corresponding diagnostic criteria.

The DSM-V is important to ensure uniformity in the approach to assessing and diagnosing mental health disorders. For instance, a lot of people believe that just feeling sad is the full equivalent of depression. However, there are more criteria required for a person to be diagnosed clinically with depression besides the feeling of sadness.

Mental health disorders for both adults and children are categorized and listed in the DSM-V.

Below are some of the categories of Mental Disorders that are Listed in the DSM-V (this is not the full list)

- Schizophrenia Spectrum and other Psychotic Disorders
- Catatonia
- Bipolar and Related Disorders
- Depressive Disorders
- Anxiety Disorders
- Obsessive-Compulsive and Related Disorders
- Trauma and Stressor Related Disorders
- Dissociative Disorders

- Somatic Symptom and Related Disorders
- Feeding and Eating Disorders
- Gender Dysphoria
- Substance-Related and Addictive Disorders
- Neurocognitive Disorders
- Personality Disorders

Every category and the disorders associated with each are clearly defined in the DSM-V. The DSM-V is under the authority of The American Psychiatric Association (APA), and they are responsible for revisions, and the guidelines outlined in the current DSM.

Mental Health Professionals

The term "mental health professional" is extremely broad, so I wanted to list some of the titles that are typically used by individuals that offer mental health services.

Mental health professionals include licensed therapist, psychologist, psychiatric nurse, psychiatric physician assistant, psychotherapist, psychiatrist, substance abuse counselors, and clinical social worker. The academic background and training vary for distinct types of mental health professionals.

I cannot say it loud enough or often enough that it is perfectly okay for black people to seek professional mental health services. There are times and seasons and reasons in our lives that will have us going to therapy. Mental health, just like physical health, must be safeguarded and we must pay attention when our mental health is not at its best.

Often, we will feel ourselves on the verge of falling apart but we keep on going anyway. It is like driving with the infamous check engine light on, ignoring it until you end up with a blown head gasket and a car that now needs major repairs. We cannot and should not ignore signs that we need to address our mental health.

Professional mental healthcare services can take many different forms. The type of professional you see, the setting, and the frequency can vary from person to person. Sadly, those with full time jobs sometimes do not have adequate coverage that will allow them to see a mental health provider without spending a lot out of pocket, which is not feasible for a lot of people.

In the world of mental health, there are various kinds of providers. I will make a brief list and try to explain the several types of providers that offer services.

Psychiatrist – This is a medical doctor (MD or DO), and they can diagnose and treat the symptoms of mental health disorders and provide medication to help their clients get their symptoms under control. Individuals experiencing any symptoms of psychosis or other serious mental health-related disorders need to visit a psychiatrist.

Psychologist – This is typically an individual that has a PhD or a PsyD and they are trained to diagnose mental health disorders and provide various forms of talk therapy to help their clients adjust to their circumstances in a healthy way.

I see people confuse the roles of psychiatrists and psychologists, and this could be due to the spelling of these words. However, these two professionals are not the same in training or function. As mentioned above, a psychiatrist (MD, DO) is a medical doctor that is specifically trained to diagnose and treat mental health disorders. They can diagnose and offer treatment, which can include medication.

Psychologists do not have the training or authority to prescribe medication, but they are able to assess, diagnose, and treat mental health disorders using various clinical techniques (e.g., cognitive behavioral therapy, positive psychology) to address the presenting issues. Currently, there are about five states that also allow psychologists (PhD, PsyD) to complete post doctorate training that will allow them to prescribe medication under the supervision of a physician. Lastly, please know that your primary care physician can also prescribe medication for mental health-related concerns.

Licensed Therapist – This is usually someone that has at least a master's degree and is licensed by their state. They can provide talk therapy in their area of focus or specialty (e.g., marriage and family).

Licensed Clinical Social Worker – This is an individual that typically has at least a master's degree in social work. They can be seen in a variety of settings and roles including offering therapy to individuals.

Substance abuse counselors, peer coaches, and other individuals also play a role in the area of mental health. I wanted to share some of the different options to help people have a better understanding of the types of professionals available to provide mental health services.

Stop Suffering in Silence

Family secrets, unresolved trauma, the death of loved ones, fertility issues, divorce, parenting challenges, addiction, and relationship struggles are a just a few reasons why people should consider going to counseling. The false narrative that we (black people) do not need counseling, and that we are strong and super-resilient has had so many black people suffer in silence unnecessarily.

For some reason, going to counseling is seen by some individuals as a sign of weakness, but getting help is not a sign of weakness; it is a sign of strength. We should want to see black men and women go to therapy more than to see them "check out" mentally one day. The people that many drive by and see as just bums or "crazy" were not born that way. People need a voice and a safe place to unpack their trauma, challenges, and heartaches so that they can heal. Overall, we do not know what someone else has endured in this journey that we call life; but one thing I do know is being kind and less judgmental is easy to do, and it is free of charge.

One thing that I want you to take away is that it is important for people to recognize the benefits of therapy. It is exciting to see more black people embracing therapy, especially black men. However, I hope that people do not treat therapy like going to the hair salon or to the barbershop. I have seen where some people are in therapy, and they enjoy going but they also express that they are not seeing any change or progress. It is important to find the right kind of therapist so that you can see the benefits of going to therapy. Every therapist does not have the same training or expertise/specialty. Ensure that you find a therapist that can assist you with your issues so that you can make progress. Liking your therapist as a person while seeing no progress is not a win. Your therapist is not your new best friend; their job is to help you improve the state of your mental health and reach your goals and objectives.

Overcoming Stigma

There are some major stigmas in the black community when it comes to mental health, and there is a lot of bad information and myths that need to be addressed. Professional mental health counseling in some cases is still frowned upon. Seeking help for your mental health can be associated with weakness and it can still be stigmatized in our families and communities.

The opinion and perception of others can be important in a lot of black and minority communities/families. I have seen this become a hindrance, and it has kept many people from getting the help that they needed. This becomes more complicated when you add being black along with being a person of faith. Many times, the same stigma in the black community carries over to the predominantly black faith communities, more specifically the predominantly black church. In certain sects of the church, symptoms of mental and physical health issues can be over-spiritualized and seen only through the lens of spirituality with no regards for physiological health, undiagnosed/untreated mental health disorders, vitamin deficiencies, sleep issues, trauma, and other factors. This means that in some cases, people are expected to pray and praise with no further recourse. The notion that mental health issues or physical health issues are indicative of a lack of faith, prayer, and trust in God are also problematic beliefs that have been perpetuated in some churches. However, there are an increasing number of efforts in various church communities to educate church leaders and congregants on mental health, and mental health first aid.

Overall, the lack of understanding regarding mental health in the black community and in the black church is still problematic. It is important because some individuals are not prone or quick to seek advice outside of those around them. This is why there is a need for our people in the secular and religious communities to be educated about some basics of mental health, including how to respond when there is a mental health crisis. Knowing how to respond in an emergency mental health situation is important.

I can say that over the past few years, the black community and the church have become more open to conversations and the normalization of counseling and getting professional mental health treatment, but there is still much work to do.

I cannot tell you how many times single black mothers have reached out to me "for a friend" because they are too scared to go to counseling. Many of these women knew that they needed help, but they were petrified that if they received services, this would lead to their children being removed from the home. Situations taken out of context and bad information that is prevalent in our communities help to fuel falsehoods like this one.

Overall, as a people we must acknowledge the trauma and great travesties of the past while highlighting the challenges of today. I cannot overemphasize the importance of mental health. You cannot be your best if you are not at your best. If your mental health is not in a good state, it must be addressed so that you can flourish in every area of your life. Leaving your mental health issues unaddressed can impact your relationships, finances, parenting, school, work, and other areas of your life. There is no benefit in "getting the bag" (making a lot of money) if you are still broken. We have all seen people with great wealth struggle with addiction, or eating disorders, succumb to suicide, or snap and commit heinous crimes – or both.

I am adamant on ensuring that people acknowledge the fact that mental health is health. Do yourself a favor and prioritize your health, and that must include your mental health!

Chapter 8.
Can Stress Affect Your Mental Health?

The topic of stress was discussed a few chapters ago. In that chapter, the body's stress response and the dangers of prolonged stress were discussed. The negative impact that stress can have on your physical health was also mentioned. In this chapter, we will look at how stress can have an impact on your mental health.

This topic is important because a lot of people have been under a lot of stress for so long that it has become normal. If you ask them to identify various sources of stress, they might not be able to recognize them because they have managed everything for so long.

Stress is not only bad for your physical health but also for your mental health. Although many of us have experienced it for what seems like our entire lives, it is not normal. As human beings we were not meant to be under stress nonstop without a break.

Just like stress can take a toll on the body, it can take a toll on the mind. Although as human beings we are a beautiful creation, we still have limitations, frailties, and weaknesses. This is so important to understand because as black people too often we are just expected to "suck it up" and keep going. The falsehood of being strong and unbreakable is still perpetuated but many times we are not seen as what we truly are; we are fragile and vulnerable like everyone else. As a black woman I cannot tell you how tired I am of this false "strong black woman" label that is always thrown around. So many black women wear it like a badge of honor and sadly, many of our beautiful black women amid staying "strong" are dying from heart disease annually. They are battling elevated levels of stress on their own while still trying to make it happen.

This is a brief list of potential sources of stress. The cause of stress will vary from one person to the next along with the severity.

- Being a single mother/father
  - When one parent is absent, the other parent can also become absent trying to work multiple jobs or excessive hours to provide. No one was meant to be a parent alone without support.
- Student loans and debt
- Financial struggles
- Overworking
- Racism
- Family turmoil and chaos
- Divorce
- Parenting
- Trauma
- Lack of sleep
- Illness
- Being a caretaker
- Relying on public transportation/No vehicle
- Living in a neighborhood with a lot of violence and crime
- Lack of upward mobility
- Poverty

Ways that stress can impact mental health

The longer you deal with chronic stress, the more at risk you are for experiencing mental health problems. Stress can lead to issues with sleep, anxiety, depression, or a mental health crisis such as a mental breakdown or suicidal ideation.[1-2] Chronic stress can also be associated with substance use/abuse which can have a major effect on a person's health and can lead to a vicious cycle of criminal behavior.

One study suggested that black males experience a greater amount of stress and that they have a higher risk for depression.[2] This is why I am a strong proponent of black males receiving professional mental health services. I have lost count of the number of black males that have stated on podcasts, blogs and so on that they have no safe space to share their hurt and pain. This is unacceptable to me, and I am glad to see an increase in podcasts, magazines, events, therapists, and counseling agencies that specialize in serving black males.

Black Mental Health Statistics

According to SAMHSA's 2020 National Survey on Drug Use and Health:

1. 17.3% (5.3 million) of Black and African American people reported having a mental illness, and 27.1% of those (1.4 million people) reported a serious mental illness.

2. Serious mental illness (SMI) rose among all ages of Black and African American people between 2008 and 2020.

3. Despite rates being less than the overall U.S. population, major depressive episodes increased from 9% to 10.3% in Black and African American youth ages twelve to seventeen; from 6.1% to 9.4% in young adults eighteen to twenty-five, and from 5.7% to 6.3% in the twenty-six to forty-nine age range between 2015 and 2020.

4. Suicidal thoughts, plans and attempts are also rising among Black and African American young adults.

5. Binge drinking, smoking (cigarettes and marijuana), illicit drug use and prescription pain reliever misuse are more frequent among Black and African American adults with mental illnesses.

These statistics should help us recognize the need to promote and have conversations about mental health in the black community. And once we have those conversations, the next step must be encouraging professional mental health services.

Finding ways to address stress in our lives is important, and our lives depend on it. Our physical and mental health are both suffering from the excess stress seen with our people. The black community is coming to the point that we are throwing off the "stay strong and show no emotion capes," we are acknowledging stress, and we are learning the importance of keeping our stress levels down as much as possible. For the sake of my own mental health, I have learned, and I am still learning to stop getting "stressed out" over things that I cannot change and are outside of my control.

Chapter References

1. Azza, Y., Grueschow, M., Karlen, W., Seifritz, E., & Kleim, B. (2020). How stress affects sleep and mental health: nocturnal heart rate increases during prolonged stress and interacts with childhood trauma exposure to predict anxiety. *Sleep, 43*(6)https://doi.org/10.1093/sleep/zsz310

2. King KM, Key-Hagan M, Desai A, et al. Stress Correlates Related to Depressive Symptoms Among Young Black Men in Southern California. *American Journal of Men's Health*. 2022;16(3). doi:10.1177/15579883221097801

Chapter 9.
Trauma

Trauma has become a buzzword over the past few years - a buzzword that some people have been using to build their brands and gain an audience. Trauma is not something that is cute and fun; trauma can be serious and has crippled the lives of many.

My definition of trauma is: "a disturbing event that is experienced or witnessed that is so distressing that the brain is impacted." Yes, it is a scientific fact that trauma can affect the human brain. Trauma can look different from one person to another. I do want to dig into this topic a little because as the topic of trauma has become more popular, people have begun to label any unpleasant event as "trauma." Everything unpleasant in life or everything we do not like or enjoy is not necessarily a traumatic event or a trigger.

PTSD

Post Traumatic Stress Disorder (PTSD) can result from a person experiencing or witnessing a very disturbing or distressing event.

Trauma can affect a person for the rest of their lives. The symptoms of PTSD can be distressing and will range in severity from person to person. PTSD can be associated with flashbacks, nightmares (of the event or something like the event), intrusive memories/thoughts, avoidant behaviors to avoid any reminders of the event, irritability, substance use/abuse, hypervigilance, changes in sleeping pattern, and difficulty concentrating.

Possible Traumatic Experiences (this list is not exhaustive)

- Sexual abuse/assault including incest
- Rape (including incest) that results in pregnancy
- Foster care
- Incarceration
- Witnessing extreme violence (shootings, stabbings)
- Finding a dead body
- Divorce
- Death of a close loved one (parent/child etc.)
- Miscarriage and stillbirth
- Financial ruin
- Homelessness (living on the streets)
- Physical abuse
- Verbal and Emotional abuse
- Extreme poverty
- Living in homes infested with rats, roaches, etc.
- Living with a hoarder
- Neglect and abandonment as a child
- Loss of all family/no family
- One or more absent parent(s)
- Incarcerated parent(s)
- Parents given lengthy prison sentences, including life
- Witnessing a loved one dying (hospice, victim of murder, etc.)
- Domestic violence in the home
- Being forced to aid parents with substance abuse (helping prepare needles and paraphernalia, etc.)

- Being put out at age eighteen with no money or support
- Losing custody of children
- Food scarcity in the home/hiding food/stealing food to avoid hunger
- Abandoned by spouse and left behind with children
- Emptied accounts/no financial support
- Death of a child
- Child(ren) missing, kidnapped by strangers or the other parent
- Diagnosed with terminal illness
- Major car accident or near-death experience
- War/military combat

Trauma can affect a person for the rest of their lives.

When seeking professional help for the aftermath of a traumatic experience, it is important to find a mental health professional that is trained and specializes in trauma. Not everyone specializes in trauma, and the purpose of seeking professional mental health services is to meet your goal of getting better and not just being able to say that you have a therapist. Mental health professionals, like physical health practitioners, have specialties. You go to a cardiologist for heart-related issues, not an OB/Gyn. So, with mental health, ensure that you find the most qualified individuals to provide the best care for your mental health concerns. Going to therapy is a good start, but for optimal results find a therapist that has the right training and experience.

Chapter 10.
Black Children + Mental Health

Children should be seen and not heard. That was a terrible mantra to live by as a parent. I cannot fathom how many children were left broken because they had no voice. Now in 2023 I do not hear that statement anymore, but a lot of children still do not have a voice. Some of those same children also do not have adults in their life that are intentional about their mental health.

I am not sure if you have been seeing studies, news reports or online articles related to the mental health of children, but a lot of children need help. The mental health of children is of major concern. Sometimes as parents it is unclear if we are in tune with or fully aware of our child's mental health. I wonder how many black kids were "whooped" for poor grades while having undiagnosed learning disorders. Or how many were punished for "out of control" behavior and acting out when they were traumatized and victims of abuse.

The mental health of children is especially important because certain issues will follow them into adulthood. For a long time, it was perpetuated that kids will just "grow out of it." A child with anxiety is not just going to grow out of it; they need professional services to address what is happening to them. If not, issues with anxiety can follow them into adulthood.

Let us look at some things that might have an impact on a child's mental health.

- Abuse of any kind
- Absent parent(s)
- Negligent parents
- Incarcerated parent(s)
- Deceased parent(s)
- Foster care
- Adoption
- Unstable housing
- Food scarcity
- Violent neighborhood
- Witnessing violence
- Being forced to commit crimes
- Being given drugs and alcohol
- Lack of basic necessities (clean clothing, bed, combed hair, clean shoes, winter coat, etc.)

Drugs and alcohol are an important topic, and I really hope that more school districts begin to train elementary and middle school staff to recognize the signs of substance use/abuse in children. I do not believe that people understand how many children are using heroin, methamphetamine and drinking hard liquor in elementary school.

Children + Mental Health

Mental health concerns in children can look quite different from mental health concerns in adults. I have seen a lot of videos of parents thinking that children are playing games to get out of school when they state that they have headaches or stomach aches. Now it is a known fact that kids will make up excuses to get out of going to school. However, in some cases, headaches and stomachaches could be an indication that something else is going on with a child.

Anxiety is one the most diagnosed mental health issues in children. Headaches and stomachaches are symptoms that can be associated with anxiety in children. Sadly, a lot of children do not get the mental health services that they need because parents might not be able to recognize mental health issues with their child. Additionally, a child is usually unable to recognize their own need for mental health services.

Here is a list of some symptoms that could be seen in a child that is dealing with potential mental health issues.

- Feelings of sadness for two weeks or more
- Isolation
- Desiring to hurt themselves or others
- Self-injurious behavior
- Suicidal ideation
- Irritability
- Drastic changes in mood, behavior, or personality
- Increase or decrease in eating
- Sudden/Unexpected loss of weight
- Sleep problems
- Frequent headaches or stomachaches
- Challenges with attentiveness and concentration
- Decrease in academic performance
- Truancy

Child Traumatic Stress + ADHD

Child traumatic stress and ADHD both have symptomology that overlap. The more trauma is understood, the more its impacts can be realized. Child traumatic stress is the term used to describe the aftermath of a traumatic experience in children. While Attention-deficit/hyperactivity disorder (ADHD) is a neurodevelopmental disorder characterized by inattention and hyperactivity-impulsivity that can impact functioning or development. Because child traumatic stress disorder has overlapping symptoms with ADHD it is important that trauma is ruled out to ensure that the correct mental health treatment is received.

Symptoms that can be seen in both ADHD and Child Traumatic Stress

- Difficulty with concentration
- Academic Issues
- Hyperactive
- Disorganized
- Sleep Problems
- Restlessness
- Distracted very easily

Symptoms of Child Traumatic Stress

- Irritability
- Easily angered
- Extremely aggressive or destructive behavior
- Disassociation
- Avoidance
- Hyperarousal

- Easily Startled

Some Symptoms of ADHD in Children

- Excessive Talking
- Difficult staying focused
- Interrupting others
- Struggles with following instructions
- Impulsiveness

Black children are believed to be more unlikely to receive professional mental health services. Some black children are at risk when they do not receive necessary treatment due to; lack of insurance that will cover services, stigma/false beliefs, or the need is not recognized or miscategorized.

The state of many of our black youth in America should give reason for us to recognize the need to prioritize and promote professional mental health counseling.

Chapter 11.
Self-Care

Self-care means many things to many people, but for the sake of simplicity we will define it as taking care of yourself. Self-care, like many other things, has become a hot topic and can be found as a hashtag on most social media platforms. Everywhere on social media you will see posts about self-care being simplified to a glass of wine and a bubble bath. Although some chose to wind down with a bubble bath and a glass of wine, I think we will miss the fullness of self-care if we limit it to those things.

The ability and act of caring for oneself will impact every aspect of our lives. This means being intentional in caring for our entire being. Self-care includes limiting external factors that cause us harm - such as recognized sources of stress, worry, and anxiety. Self-care does not imply escapism or trying to avoid any hardships or negative factors in life, but it does mean making our total health a priority and not neglecting ourselves.

Self-care means not running your body to the ground, trying to work twenty-three hours per day and survive off one hour of sleep. You have the right to rest and should not feel that you will miss "the bag" if you get a good night's rest. I am a believer of whatever is for me, is for me, so in the meantime I am going to get some good rest because I need and deserve to rest.

Self-Care + Mothers

Self-care is so important for black people, especially mothers, as we give so much and do so much. Working, cooking, cleaning, school, business, taking care of the kids and everything else can be a lot over time, especially if you are carrying the load alone. I was a single mother for years and I can recognize how much I neglected myself. Sometimes you need to take some time to decompress and just relax. You might need to take a day and do absolutely nothing but rest, or you can do something that you enjoy.

Take time to do things that you love and enjoy. Take time to be truly gentle with yourself and love yourself. How often have we been more concerned and caring about others while overlooking our own needs? Now this is not a call to neglect our responsibilities as adults, but it is a gentle reminder that in the grand scheme of things, do not forget about you.

Protecting Yourself

Self-care can include the introduction of healthy boundaries or limitations in our lives. Boundaries can help you avoid unnecessary drama, headaches, and heartaches. How many times have you allowed people a front row seat in your life too quickly? How often have you allowed people to pressure you into things that you did not want to do? Boundaries can help protect your peace, your heart, your finances, and your energy. Boundaries can serve different purposes for different kinds of relationships and people in our lives. Setting boundaries can mean not allowing people to have access to you all day, every day. It can also mean not allowing people to come in and out of your life as they please.

Boundaries can mean saying no and not allowing people to pressure, bully, or guilt-trip you into things that you do not want to do while neglecting ourselves. Now, I am a firm believer in serving others and using my life to be a blessing to other people. However, I will not run myself down while helping others and forsaking myself. Being able to prioritize and having some sense of "balance" and order is important.

Take care of yourself because you will depend on you for your entire lifetime. Love yourself because you deserve as much love and grace as you give to others. Be gentle with yourself; you deserve as much understanding as you give to others. Amid all the busyness and bustle of life, make sure you take care of yourself.

Pick up old hobbies or start new ones; go to therapy, work on your physical health, travel, and do things that you love and enjoy. We have one life to live, so live well. And if money is tight remember resting, logging out of social media, and taking time to just exist doesn't require you to spend any money.

If we are to call ourselves truly "woke" or conscious (aware), then we must become aware of the state of black health. -D'Andrea Bolden, MA

Spirit.
Spiritual Health

To date there is no standard and widely accepted definition for spiritual health. I define spiritual health as connecting with God (Creator), the realization of life beyond the physical, living out one's purpose and helping others to do the same.

Intro

As a black Christian woman, I can say that on a large scale, a lot of black people have been around various religions and belief systems since they were kids. But in many cases, we do not see our people as spiritually healthy and in a state of peace. We are never taught to rest, relax, and incorporate spiritual practices in a way that contributes positively to our overall health.

Many of us were introduced to various belief systems during times of environmental, financial, family, and internal chaos. Some grew up only seeing the family turn to religion and spirituality due to the hardships of life, which skewed their view because they might have never seen religion or spirituality without a crisis. Sadly, misconceptions about faith in God and personal responsibility have left a bad taste in the mouth of many individuals.

With that said, in this section I am going to discuss various spiritual practices and the science that supports how they can be beneficial to one's health overall (holistic).

Chapter 12.
Spiritual Health: Prayer

Prayer, like many other spiritual practices, is quite old. For some, it is tradition, and for others, it is dedication or duty. Prayer is something that many of us were taught to do as children. I am sure that you are aware that we live in a world where people ascribe to a variety of religious and spiritual beliefs, and chances are, a sizable number of these people believe in prayer. The way a person approaches prayer, the reasons for prayer, and how often they pray can vary greatly. In fact, some people are taught to pray at certain times of the day, on specific days of the week, and in certain locations.

Prayer is incredibly significant to a nation when there is a holiday called The National Day of Prayer. This holiday was first signed into law by then acting President Harry S. Truman in 1952. It is a day that the citizens of the USA are suggested to pray and meditate and focus on God. Although everyone does not associate with a particular religious or spiritual path, some still feel the "call" to pray.

Some individuals pray to feel connected and commune with the god of their (religion) faith, while some without a particular belief system pray to acknowledge a higher power or their creator.

There are several studies that suggest prayer might have some benefits. I mentioned that because someone who is reading this book might not be connected to any belief system and they might question the reasons that other people pray.

VanderWeele, Balboni, and Koh (2017) shared that studies have suggested there is a casual association with attending religious services and a lowered risk of depression.[3] They also shared that person-centered medical care could benefit from including a focus on spirituality, however more research is needed on more diverse populations.[3]

Behavioral scientists have had discussions about whether prayer should be considered an alternative form of medicine. Yet, the inability to present a biomedical explanation for any effects attributed to prayer would hinder them from coming to this conclusion. They cannot prove, using their standards and scientific protocols, that prayer works and that it makes a measurable and reproducible impact. Prayer, like many other aspects of spirituality and spiritual health, will not meet the rigorous requirement for validation and acceptance by the scientific community.

Spirituality goes beyond the physical, which is why the ability to use science to explain and collect data can get complicated and, in some cases, it can be impossible. But this does not and will not stop people from believing and having faith. There is a Scripture that I believe gives a great definition of faith.

> Now faith is confidence in what we hope for and assurance about what we do not see. (*Hebrews 11:1, NIV*)

Faith plays a role in spiritual health because many of the practices that people engage in, such as prayer, are things that they strongly believe in and live by. The spiritual beliefs and practices of many people are ancient and pre-date modern science. This truth does not invalidate science, nor does the truth of science invalidate spirituality. But it does mean that these are two distinct components of life.

Prayer should not always be focused on oneself, but we should pray on behalf of others. This is known as intercessory prayer. When we pray in faith, we expect to see the outcome for that which we prayed. We believe that God is almighty to respond to our righteous requests that agree with His written Word. When I was taught how to pray, one of the first things I was taught was how to pray the Scriptures back to the Lord. So, below I have shared a few Scriptures.

> Therefore I tell you, whatever you ask in prayer, believe that you have received it, and it will be yours. **(Mark 11:24, ESV)**

> Therefore, confess your sins to one another and pray for one another, that you may be healed. The prayer of a righteous person has great power as it is working. **(James 5:16, ESV)**

In my personal life, prayer is something that I practice on a regular basis. I pray to commune with the Lord, make my petitions and requests known, and release my burdens. Prayer is a form of expression, and it allows us to release and verbalize our internal concerns.

Do not be anxious about anything, but in every situation, by prayer and petition, with thanksgiving, present your requests to God. (*Philippians 4:6, NIV*)

...praying at all times in the Spirit, with all prayer and supplication. To that end, keep alert with all perseverance, making supplication for all the saints... (*Ephesians 6:18, ESV*)

And whatever we ask we receive from him, because we keep his commandments and do what pleases him. (*I John 3:22, ESV*)

And this is the confidence that we have toward him, that if we ask anything according to his will he hears us. (*I John 5:14, ESV*)

Pray without ceasing. (*I Thessalonians 5:17, KJV*)

And whatever you ask in prayer, you will receive, if you have faith." (*Matthew 21:22, ESV*)

...casting all your anxieties on him because he cares for you – (*I Peter 5:7, ESV*)

Although science does not support the benefits of prayer with evidence, people all around the globe believe in the power of prayer. People pray about things that are affecting their physical and mental health. They pray about the things that are happening in and to their lives. When people pray, they have faith that their prayers will be answered. Are all prayers answered the way that people expect? The answer to that is no, just like every attempt of science and medicine to solve a problem is not always successful.

Overall, prayer, for many like me, is a major component of our lives. I do not see prayer as a substitute to medical care or professional mental health services; however, like faith, it is a pillar to my spiritual health.

Prayer has its place, just like exercising has its place in my life. Both are important and one does not replace the other. Prayer is an important aspect of our spiritual health, and our spiritual health is a significant component of our overall health from a holistic perspective.

Chapter References

1. VanderWeele, T. J., Balboni, T. A., & Koh, H. K. (2017). Health and spirituality. JAMA: The Journal of the American Medical Association, 318(6), 519-520. https://doi.org/10.1001/jama.2017.8136

2. Masters, K. S., & Spielmans, G. I. (2007). Prayer and health: Review, meta-analysis, and research agenda. Journal of Behavioral Medicine, 30(4), 329-338. https://doi.org/10.1007/s10865-007-9106-7

3. VanderWeele TJ, Yu J, Cozier YC, Wise L, Argentieri MA, Rosenberg L, Palmer JR, Shields AE. Attendance at Religious Services, Prayer, Religious Coping, and Religious/Spiritual Identity as Predictors of All-Cause Mortality in the Black Women's Health Study. Am J Epidemiol. 2017 Apr 1;185(7):515-522. doi: 10.1093/aje/kww179. Erratum in: Am J Epidemiol. 2017 Aug 15;186(4):501. PMID: 28338863; PMCID: PMC6354668.

Chapter 13.

Spiritual Health: Fasting

Fasting is a practice that people use for health reasons, or for religious and spiritual reasons. There are scientifically proven benefits associated with fasting, which is why a lot of people with no religious or spiritual affiliation will still participate in fasting. Not everyone fasts the same way or for the same reasons or desired outcomes, but in this book, I want to focus on fasting as a component of spiritual health.

When I refer to fasting, I am talking about fasting from food. I know people will "fast" or avoid other things such as sex, television, and other pleasures, but for the sake of simplicity I am referring only to food.

Fasting is when you do not eat for a certain period. Fasting for some people can be extremely hard, and it can take a lot of discipline. It is important to ensure that fasting does not override sound medical advice. If you must take food with your medicine, then you need to do that to avoid any consequences of not properly taking your medication.

There is research that suggests that fasting is beneficial to your health. Fasting can be done for natural and spiritual benefits. From a spiritual perspective, fasting helps to shift your focus as you make a sacrifice. It can also help with discipline and can build stamina in your spiritual walk. Fasting can also help you get a hold of your impulses and distractions especially when it is coupled with prayer, meditation, and reading of the Scriptures.

Benefits of Fasting

- Helps improve blood sugar control by reducing insulin resistance
- Can combat inflammation (inflammation is believed to be the cause of the development and progression of many diseases)
- Can be beneficial to brain health
- Could be beneficial to the treatment and prevention of cancer[1]
- Can improve blood pressure, triglycerides, and cholesterol levels
- Can be helpful for weight loss
- Reduced insulin growth factor which promotes cell death

Intermittent fasting is believed to have several benefits listed above, according to the Mayo Clinic. With intermittent fasting you restrict food intake for certain periods of time, and you eat during the time you are not restricting food intake. There are several distinct types of fasting. Before you start, it is important to speak with your provider before attempting any extreme or long-term fasting. I have seen multiple people get sick from fasting and not taking their medication or attempting an extreme form of fasting. Let us be wise and get sound professional medical advice before fasting.

Chapter References

1. Clifton, K. K., Ma, C. X., Fontana, L., & Peterson, L. L. (2021). Intermittent fasting in the prevention and treatment of cancer. *CA: a cancer journal for clinicians, 71*(6), 527–546. https://doi.org/10.3322/caac.21694

Chapter 14.

Spiritual Health: Meditation

Over the past few decades, we have seen an increase in people practicing meditation, being more health conscious, and promoting self-care. Meditation, like prayer, is an ancient practice that predates modern science. Meditation is practiced all around the world by people that are associated with various religions and spiritual belief systems and those that are non-religious and non-spiritual.

Typically seen as an Eastern philosophy associated with Buddhism and Hinduism, meditation has become more prevalent in Western society in a more secular form that is detached from any specific religion. The most popular form of secular meditation is referred to as mindfulness-meditation. There is a lot of research on mindfulness-based stress reduction (MBSR) which is an actual program that was created to help people that are managing pain, stress, anxiety, and illness.[1] Research has suggested that MBSR can be helpful with clinical and nonclinical related issues.[1]

Researchers typically make reference to two types of meditation - concentration meditation and mindfulness meditation.[2] The objective of concentration meditation is to focus on one thing until the mind reaches a state of quietness and is believed to help with mental clarity and relaxation.[2] Mindfulness meditation is focused on being judgment-free while being aware of one's thoughts and emotions, and it is strongly believed to help people create new ways to cope with the various issues of life.[2] Other researchers also acknowledge other forms of meditation such as transcendental meditation, loving-kindness meditation and secular meditation.[3]

Meditation has been found to be effective for some aspects of physical and mental health. It was shared that meditation can be associated with small improvements with pain, depression, stress, and anxiety.[3] Allen (2020) also expressed that although meditation can be beneficial, it is not a cure.

So, what is meditation all about? Meditation is a practice that builds discipline and focus. A lot of people are going non-stop and never take the time to slow down and be still in their mind and body because they are moving around all day. Meditation allows you to be present, intentional, and more aware of your thoughts and your environment. You can quiet yourself and notice things that you do not normally think about such as your breathing, your heart rate, and overall, how you feel from the inside out.

Based on my perspective as a Christian, my definition of meditation is the intentional contemplation and focus on God and His Word. Meditation means bringing the mind into focus on Scriptures and on the goodness of God. I cannot overemphasize how meditation is such an important aspect of spiritual health - not just for Christians, but for many people around the world.

The reason I mention meditation from a Christian perspective is that studies have shown that Christians can be opposed to meditation due to the fear of it being associated with other religious practices,[4] which leads many Christians to reject the practice of meditation in any form.

CHRISTIANS + MEDITATION

As mentioned before, meditation has become quite popular and is openly promoted. However, I want to take a moment to share what meditation looks like for those that adhere to the Christian faith. I recognize that everyone that reads this book is not a Christian and that is fine, but for those that are, I want to add this information. Consider this: although other belief systems embrace meditation, they might not approach meditation the way we would as believers in Jesus Christ.

The Bible has more than twenty Scriptures referring to meditation, but this is not something that is typically focused on in a lot of churches. This is why Christians need to know the Word and what God says in His Word about meditation.

Meditation for us is not focused on emptying our minds or focused mindfulness, or just awareness of self; instead, it includes the intentional practice of filling our minds with the Word of God.

WHAT IS MEDITATION?

Here are two Hebrew words and one Greek word for meditation:

1. **hâgâh (H1897) *haw-gaw'***

   Strong's Exhaustive Concordance – Definition: To murmur (in pleasure or anger); to ponder, imagine, meditate, mourn, mutter, roar, speak, study, talk, utter

2. **śîychâh (H7881) *see-khaw'***

Strong's Exhaustive Concordance – Definition: Reflection, devotion, meditation, prayer

3. **This is a Greek word – meletaō (G3191)** *mel-et-ah'-o*

Strong's Exhaustive Concordance – Definition: To take care of, revolve in the mind, imagine

When we meditate, we are rehearsing in our minds and pondering on God's Word, on His goodness, and on righteous things. When we meditate, there is a deliberate focus on God and His Word. We can meditate on His goodness and on righteous things because the Bible tells us to think on these things, "Finally, brothers, whatever is true, whatever is honorable, whatever is just, whatever is pure, whatever is lovely, whatever is commendable, if there is any excellence, if there is anything worthy of praise, think about these things." *(Philippians 4:8, ESV)*

II. TIPS FOR MEDITATION

Meditation is a discipline that takes time to develop, so I want to share a few tips to help you as you begin to meditate. Also, I have shared several Scriptures so that you can see what God's Word says about meditation.

1. Find Scriptures to rehearse and ponder.

2. Find Scriptures to memorize.

3. Find Scriptures to pray back to the Lord.

4. Think of His goodness, His greatness, His presence, etc.

5. Be intentional in focusing your mind on God, His Word, etc.

6. Do not give up when you lose focus; just refocus your mind again.

7. Grab a journal and pen to write after you have spent time meditating.

8. Do not rush!! Meditation is not something that you rush to do in thirty seconds, so take your time.

III. SCRIPTURES FOR MEDITATION

This Book of the Law shall not depart from your mouth, but you shall meditate on it day and night, so that you may be careful to do according to all that is written in it. For then you will make your way prosperous, and then you will have good success. **(Joshua 1:8, ESV)**

Let the words of my mouth and the meditation of my heart be acceptable in your sight, O Lord, my rock and my redeemer. **(Psalm 19:14, ESV)**

...but his delight is in the law of the Lord, and on his law he meditates day and night. **(Psalm 1:2, ESV)**

I will meditate on your precepts and fix my eyes on your ways. **(Psalm 119: 15, ESV)**

May my meditation be pleasing to him, for I rejoice in the Lord. **(Psalm 104:34, ESV)**

Oh, how I love your law! It is my meditation all the day. **(Psalm 119:97, ESV)**

My mouth shall speak wisdom; the meditation of my heart shall be understanding. **(Psalm 49:3, ESV)**

...when I remember you upon my bed, and meditate on you in the watches of the night... **(Psalm 63:6, ESV)**

I remember the days of old; I meditate on all that you have done; I ponder the work of your hands. **(Psalm 143:5, ESV)**

My eyes are awake before the watches of the night, that I may meditate on your promise. **(Psalm 119:148, ESV)**

I will ponder all your work, and meditate on your mighty deeds. **(Psalm 77:12, ESV)**

I have more understanding than all my teachers, for your testimonies are my meditation. **(Psalm 119:99, ESV)**

Let the insolent be put to shame, because they have wronged me with falsehood; as for me, I will meditate on your precepts. **(Psalm 119:78, ESV)**

I will lift up my hands toward your commandments, which I love, and I will meditate on your statutes. **(Psalm 119:48, ESV)**

Even though princes sit plotting against me, your servant will meditate on your statutes. **(Psalm 119:23, ESV)**

On the glorious splendor of your majesty, and on your wondrous works, I will meditate. **(Psalm 145:5, ESV)**

I will meditate on your precepts and fix my eyes on your ways. I will delight in your statutes; I will not forget your word. **(Psalm 119:15-16, ESV)**

Chapter References

1. Grossman P, Niemann L, Schmidt S, et al. Mindfulness-based stress reduction and health benefits: a meta-analysis. 2004. In: Database of Abstracts of Reviews of Effects (DARE): Quality-assessed Reviews [Internet]. York (UK): Centre for Reviews and Dissemination (UK); 1995-. Available from: https://www.ncbi.nlm.nih.gov/books/NBK70854/]

2. Sampaio, C., Lima, M., & Ladeia, A. (2017). Meditation, Health and Scientific Investigations: Review of the Literature. Journal of Religion and Health,56 (2), 411-427. Retrieved from http://www.jstor.org/stable/44158323

3. Allen, C. (2020). The potential health benefits of meditation. ACSM's Health & Fitness Journal, 24(6), 28-32. https://doi.org/10.1249/FIT.0000000000000624

4. Woods-Giscombé, C. L., & Gaylord, S. A. (2014). The Cultural Relevance of Mindfulness Meditation as a Health Intervention for African Americans: Implications for Reducing Stress-Related Health Disparities. *Journal of Holistic Nursing, 32*(3), 147–160. https://doi.org/10.1177/0898010113519010

Chapter 15.

Spiritual Health: Affirmations

Daily affirmations can be powerful when used correctly. When we share affirmations, we are taking the time to speak something as true, or we are speaking those things that do not yet exist as if they were already manifested.

> Now faith is confidence in what we hope for and assurance about what we do not see. (*Hebrews 11:1, NIV*)

Words have the power to shift and shape your world. I once heard a saying that, "Words create worlds." The words you speak have power, and those words can affect your thinking and your behavior. If a lot of people were honest about the way they speak to themselves internally, it would be extremely negative. So, it is not a shock when those same people speak negatively in their everyday lives and to other people.

We must learn that since words are powerful, we should be careful of what we say. Words are like spiritual containers that have power and meaning. Some people cannot see the connection between a negative mind, negative words, and a negative life. Research has shown that speaking to plants can be beneficial to their growth. However, it was also discovered that speaking negatively and in an unpleasant tone does not help with growth. So, if a plant can be impacted by words, how about you? What about your life, or your marriage and children?

There might be someone reading this book who is still bothered by negative words that were spoken to them when they were a young child. They have never forgotten those words and it still bothers them to this day. Words can hurt us and haunt us because words are so powerful.

The words we speak will yield a fruitful harvest whether we like it or not. For this reason, I hate to hear people say things like they do not have money, they are a failure, or that they are unwanted - as if it is a part of their identity. The words we speak will ensnare us if we are not careful.

> Death and life are in the power of the tongue: and they that love it shall eat the fruit thereof.
> **(Proverbs 18:21, KJV)**

Think before you speak and use your mouth to create your abundant and blessed future. Many have the tendency to speak very negatively when they are angry. This can include calling themselves dumb, stupid, or even lashing out at a spouse and children. Sadly, I have lost count of mothers that have told their children that they would amount to nothing and that they would become just like their father (i.e., alcoholic, incarcerated, addict, homeless, abusive, etc.). As parents, we have the power to speak words of destiny over our children because there are far too many adults who were damaged by the words of their own parents during their childhood.

If an individual is accustomed to negativity in every aspect of life, it will take consistency and intention to get things going in the right direction. Years of toxic thinking, speaking, and behavior will not be undone overnight. The process of unlearning these things can begin by creating new habits. When I refer to habits, I am thinking about good daily practices that can be repeated. The more you implement daily affirmations, the easier repeating affirmations as a spiritual practice will become.

Examples of Daily Affirmations

- I am brilliant.
- I am successful.
- I deserve to be happy.
- I believe in myself.
- I am building a successful life.
- My children will be successful.
- Our family will prosper and lack no good thing.

My suggestion for anyone is to find affirmations that best fit the life that they are trying to create. My affirmations will be different than yours, and vice versa because we all have specific goals and objectives that we are trying to achieve. A lot of people will use positive affirmations, but personally I use a mixture of positive and biblical affirmations. Biblical affirmations mean that they correspond with specific Scriptures. I will find Scriptures and incorporate them into my affirmations.

I love affirmations as they help us speak and confess positive things. This helps us to focus mentally on what we ponder so that our actions can line up accordingly. Although I love affirmations, they do require effort on our part. You can say every day that you are going to lose weight, but if you never exercise and you now eat more than you normally do, chances are that is not going to happen.

So, we need to ensure that our actions agree with our affirmations. Some individuals are unaware that they have been speaking and affirming things all their lives, but they were mostly negative or destructive. The older I get, the more I monitor what I say out of my mouth because I know that my words have power and what I say will manifest. Speaking positively is a discipline that you must practice.

> Set a guard over my mouth, LORD; keep watch over the door of my lips. **(Psalm 141:3, NIV)**

Research on self-affirmations has shared results that suggest an increase in executive functions (organization, emotional regulation, focus), and is believed to be associated with the activation of neural reward pathways.[1-2] The activation of neural reward pathways associates the task performed with satisfaction - "reward" - and will increase your likeliness of repeating the behavior.

Chapter References

1. Harris, P. S., Harris, P. R., & Miles, E. (2017). Self-affirmation improves performance on tasks related to executive functioning. Journal of Experimental Social Psychology, 70, 281-285. https://doi.org/10.1016/j.jesp.2016.11.011

2. Dutcher, J. M., Creswell, J. D., Pacilio, L. E., Harris, P. R., Klein, W. M. P., Levine, J. M., Bower, J. E., Muscatell, K. A., & Eisenberger, N. I. (2016). Self-affirmation activates the ventral striatum: A possible reward-related mechanism for self-affirmation. Psychological Science, 27(4), 455-466. https://doi.org/10.1177/0956797615625989

Stress is a silent enemy wreaking havoc in the lives of many black people. – **D'Andrea Bolden**

Whole.

Holistic Health

Holistic health considers the whole person; it is a multidimensional and comprehensive way to consider health and wellness.

Chapter 16.
Embracing Holistic Health

When I refer to holistic health, it includes multiple factors that are a part of our total wellness or well-being. To be completely healthy (or well), we must consider all aspects of our wellness. This means not just embracing a vegan lifestyle while ignoring our mental health or exercising every day while never addressing your spiritual health. Doing that would mean that you are not addressing every aspect of your health.

Ok, because spirituality and religious beliefs can be taken to the extreme there can be a need for balance. This simply means that we should not over spiritualize things that need a natural or practical approach. Let me make that plain. As someone who grew up in the church, I have lost count of how many times people wanted to use "faith" as a reason to do nothing about practical things (i.e. illness, vocation, finances, losing weight, therapy, etc.) that should be addressed. Even the Bible states that faith without works (action) is dead (James 2:26).

As human beings, we are a spirit that lives in a body and that possesses a soul. Therefore, we must learn to take care of every part of our being to be at our best. Think about it - when a person has a physical health crisis, it could cause them to feel depressed (mental health) and as a result, they may struggle with or even lose faith (spiritual health). I found it very interesting to recognize that one component of our wellness can affect another aspect of our wellness. I wish I knew more about health, wellness, and holistic health while I was growing up. Many of us struggled and some still struggle, not realizing the importance of total health and wellness.

One thing that made me more aware was seeing the mention of body, soul, and spirit in Scripture. It was like an "aha" moment that I am more than just a body; that there is more to me, and that all of me needs to be whole, with nothing lacking.

> And the very God of peace sanctify you wholly; and *I pray God* your whole spirit and soul and body be preserved blameless unto the coming of our Lord Jesus Christ. (**I Thessalonians 5:23, KJV**)

Currently, there is still pushback against the use of alternative treatments alongside traditional methods. Some individuals see this as "quack" science and others believe that it would lead to people having less faith/seeing less value in traditional western medicine. I do not know if this is true, but I am convinced that many are simply beginning to recognize the need to treat the whole man and not just one aspect.

Researchers have shared that health goes beyond the body and they acknowledge that the soul (mind) and spirit have an effect or impact on each other.[1] Hence, this is why we should embrace holistic health to ensure that individuals are well in every aspect.

Social health should be included as well, as it emphasizes our need for belonging by having and maintaining healthy relationships and being able to handle conflict in our social relationships.

Financial wellness should be included in holistic health as well because there is a high number of black people living in poverty. We know that much of it was caused by tactics that have oppressed and robbed many of wealth. In addition, we must also recognize how poverty and financial lack can contribute to stress which, as mentioned earlier in this book, can affect a person's overall health. The rat race for a slice of the pie, never being able to get ahead, single mothers working two and three jobs, and "robbing Peter to pay Paul" takes a toll after a while. So, for black people we must consider financial security and wellness as a part of our holistic health.

There is a growing number of legitimate organizations that teach and educate our people on financial literacy, diversified income streams, building generational wealth, estate planning, life insurance, youth college funds and many other things that can help us gain our footing financially and provide some upward mobility.

Below is a list of what I consider to be the most important aspects of holistic health for black people.

Holistic health is nothing new. For years I saw a lot of people promoting holistic health and I ignored it. I did not think it was important or that it had any value. I looked at their super healthy lifestyles including their herbs and blended drinks and I laughed. Well, now that I am a bit older and wiser, I am not laughing anymore; instead, I have been learning. If many of us embraced the diet and nutrition aspects associated with holistic health and wellness, we might not have as many needs that can only be properly addressed and managed by allopathic (MD) and osteopathic (DO) medical professionals. I know some people ignore everything that their doctor tells them, and it has caused some to have their health spiral out of control unnecessarily and others departed from this earth much sooner than they should have.

Mental health is a vital aspect of holistic health and in the black community, I can say that we are making progress, and social media has been a huge help in the fight against misinformation and stigma. There are several initiatives to promote black mental health. I reflect on my childhood, and growing up I never heard the words therapist or mental health. I ponder how many black families could have been healed or individuals that could have resolved childhood trauma and other issues if we understood the importance and need to prioritize mental health. With self-care being a hot topic, some people are thinking that a glass of wine and a bubble bath is enough. Although those might help you with relaxing and winding down, they are not considered professional solutions to help you heal, equip you with tools to cope, walk you through grief and trauma, or address other pertinent mental health concerns. Self-care goes beyond cute fuzzy socks and journals. Sometimes it includes doing the work and seeing a mental health professional so that your soul can finally heal.

> Beloved, I pray that you may prosper in all things and be in health, just as your soul prospers. (**III John 1:2, NKJV**)

Ways to Embrace Holistic Health

1. Exercise
2. Healthy diet/clean eating

3. Do not ignore dietary and exercise instructions provided by your physician (low salt diet, low carb diet, exercise 30 minutes daily, etc.)
4. Regular physicals and checkups
5. Follow all the instructions from your physician
6. Proper dental care
7. Consider professional mental health counseling for any of the following:
    a. Childhood trauma
    b. Stress
    c. Anxiety
    d. Depression
    e. Anger and unforgiveness
    f. Suicidal thoughts
    g. Hallucinations
    h. Delusions
    i. Abuse
    j. Any other reason that you feel you need to go
8. Family and marriage counseling
    a. Marital issues
    b. Blended families
    c. Child-parent conflict
    d. Stepchild-stepparent conflict
    e. Unhealthy family dynamics
    f. Any other reason you feel you need to go
9. Self-care
    a. Rest
    b. Stay hydrated
    c. Boundaries
    d. Prioritizing all the people and things in your life
10. Meditation

11. Prayer
12. Affirmations
13. Fasting
14. Buildup your faith
15. Build healthy relationships
16. Learn effective communication
17. Financial literacy
18. Get help to get out of debt
19. Be a good financial steward
20. Find resources to assist with financial literacy and security.
21. Anything else important to you

I believe that now, more than ever before, it is imperative that black people all around the world begin to prioritize their health on all levels. It is also necessary that we become educated and informed so that we can help our children, so that the next generation is not left clueless.

We can reach the younger generation by introducing them to physical activities and exercise, educating them about nutrition, teaching them about finances, teaching them about healthy relationships, and explaining the importance of mental health. Overall, I believe that we can make great strides individually and collectively if we all begin to invest in our holistic health.

Chapter References

1. Patwardhan, B., Matali, G., & Tillu, G. (2015, April 10). *Concepts of health and disease*. Integrative Approaches for Health. Retrieved from https://www.sciencedirect.com/science/article/pii/B978012801 2826000036.

Chapter 17.

Embracing Rest For Your Health

I know many people are asking when did living off a few hours of sleep and grinding non-stop become the norm and the thing to do? Why are we treating self-neglect like some badge of honor that we should all be working towards? I get it; you must work hard to get anything in this world. But is it worth your health? We have the tendency to not value our health until illness comes along.

Our bodies get tired and need rest for a reason. Some people might need more rest than others. Yet others might have health-related issues that cause fatigue. At the end of the day, if you feel tired, it is okay to skip energy drinks and get some sleep. I know we live in a culture where many treat sleep deprivation as a required benchmark on the road to success.

Like an alarm or warning light in our car, we should never ignore the needs of our bodies, and this includes sleep. Instead, our mindset should be ensuring that we give our bodies the rest and nutrients required because we need our body and mind to be healthy. We must normalize taking care of the body and mind that we need throughout our earthly journey. With that said, there is no shame in taking a break from unnecessary busy activities, logging out of social media, setting a bedtime if necessary, and setting boundaries so that people are not draining you.

I have always been told that success comes in the form of good daily habits. That means that I do not have to get only three hours of sleep every day and drag my body and mind down the toilet to become successful. Health, like many other things, is not missed until it is gone. You can protect your health today by getting enough rest and by learning to relax. I know it is not always easy, but trust me, if you knew that neglecting your body would lead to bad health down the road, I am quite sure that you would make changes today. Some people become successful at the expense of their own health and are unable to enjoy the fruit of their labor.

Rest is good for mental health and clarity, but there are many other benefits associated with getting enough rest. I want to share some of the scientifically proven benefits of rest on your physical and mental health.

Researchers have shared that a lack of sleep can lead to several health issues such as heart disease, kidney disease, high blood pressure, diabetes, stroke, and obesity.[1] The National Sleep Foundation stated that adults between ages eighteen to sixty-four should sleep seven to nine hours per night.[2] They also shared that older adults who are sixty-five and older should typically sleep between seven to eight hours per night.[1]

If someone reading this is having sleeping issues you need to talk to your doctor as soon as possible so they can ensure that you are not experiencing a physical or mental health issue that requires intervention (diagnosis and treatment). Some physicians will recommend a sleep study to better understand any potential issues.

Chapter References

1.   Lichtenstein G. R. (2015). The Importance of Sleep. *Gastroenterology & hepatology, 11*(12), 790.

Chapter 18.
Professional Integrative Care

Hopefully, the information from the other chapters has helped you understand holistic health a little better. This chapter will discuss what mental health and medical professionals can do to help you improve your holistic health.

Although I am a proponent of holistic health to be at your best, I am not a proponent of fake internet gurus, self-proclaimed experts or snake oil salespeople convincing the masses that they have the "cure." Recently I saw people online wanting to become practitioners of natural medicine with no formal education from an accredited university. This is troublesome, as no one's health should be put in the hands of an untrained individual. While spirituality, nutrition, and diet have a place in holistic health, they are not a replacement for professional healthcare. We still need to understand and value the role of primary care physicians and mental health practitioners.

Observing unbalanced perspectives from others in their quest for "health" is one of the reasons why I shunned holistic health for years. Many like to overemphasize certain aspects of holistic health - such as the spiritual side - along with unverified remedies. At the same time, people will forego professional medical advice and cease professional medical treatment, which can be extremely dangerous. I have seen too many people hospitalized due to throwing out all of their medication and trying to treat their own health conditions. You should always work with your physician to ensure that your efforts are not causing more harm than good. We should not see trained professionals as the enemy or a blockade to total health. A working relationship is important because while many aspects of a holistic health approach are beneficial, when a person has a physical disease or mental health disorder, they should always seek professional care.

It bothers me that many times black people are the target of so much misinformation because the internet is used heavily by predators that know some of us are not well-versed in the sciences and do not know much about health. These predators also play on the fact that many black people mistrust and are dissatisfied with white practitioners and traditional western medicine, and they use that distrust to gain trust with minorities and deceive people for their own financial gain.

Some of the things I see on social media are so farfetched it is beyond shocking that people fall for it. In many cases, if people would do a quick Google search or call a board-certified physician, they would find out quickly that these people are making false claims and getting fake reviews to make themselves seem credible to make money and build an audience. Yes, fake reviews to build a profitable platform is a real thing, so be discerning on the internet.

I said all that to say that your health is invaluable, so please do not put your health in the hands of someone that is not qualified. I do not want to see anyone, especially those with a terminal illness or a chronic disease, putting their hopes in something on the internet that could be false, cause their health to decline at a faster pace, or lead to unnecessary complications. Individuals should not be placing other lives in jeopardy by trying to become popular or make sales.

There is a reason why medical and mental health professionals go through years of academia and training. There must be standards to minimize harm to people seeking treatment. It is very risky to seek help from someone that is not a state-licensed mental health professional or a board-certified physician. There are consequences that come along with taking such a risk.

People will see someone promoting something as a "cure" or read testimonials and get excited. They will then jump on the bandwagon to try out this alleged "cure." Even if their claims are true, you might not have the same results. Why? Because you could have more health issues or a more chronic health issue. Their diet and lifestyle could be quite different from yours. Therefore, seeking cures while ignoring professional medical advice can be disastrous; in fact, some people have died.

With this book, my goal was to present the information to you. I have made zero medical claims, and I am not promoting cures, nor am I pushing or promoting any health-related products for you to take.

Integrative Medicine

Over the years there has been more research, and more practitioners that are in favor of integrative or preventative care. This can be an approach for both physiological and mental health. A lot of people want more than traditional care; instead, they want treatment that considers their total being: body, mind (soul), and spirit.

Did you know that there is an increased demand in hospitals from patients wanting integrative medical care? Integrative medicine is being evaluated as a potential solution to help with the overwhelming issues plaguing the American healthcare system. Integrative medicine is poised to be patient-centered and healing-oriented due to the emphasis on treating the whole person and not just symptoms.

I cannot over-emphasize the importance of receiving all medical care from a board-certified medical professional. I want to ensure no one walks away from this book thinking that I would ever endorse you putting your health and your life in the hands of someone that is not a trained professional. Integrative medical care should be in coordination with a licensed medical professional. I must emphasize this because sometimes people can misconstrue what is being communicated, so hopefully this clears up any misconception that someone might have had.

Integrative Mental Healthcare

Many in the professional community have become more aware of the demand for integrative mental healthcare. In fact, there is a push for standardized research, education, and an evidence-supported model for integrative mental healthcare that can be utilized in a clinical setting.[4]

Why is this important? For example, some individuals with mental health issues are dealing with comorbidity. Comorbidity refers to multiple disorders at the same time. Some people are dealing with mental health issues and physical health conditions or even a substance use disorder.[2] Comorbidity can make treatment more complex and this can affect an individual's response to treatment.[2] Researchers also shared that there are some notable limitations to a traditional approach, especially with psychiatric care.[2-3] Some have advocated for the merging of the bio-psycho-social-spiritual model with alternative healing practices such as herbs, meditation, and acupuncture.[4] Alternative healing practices would be in addition to any pharmacologic treatments, psychotherapy, and psychosocial interventions.[4]

One thing that I hope I have made clear is that integrative care is defined as the inclusion of alternative/ non-traditional methods in addition to more traditional evidence-based treatments. The world of health, science, and medicine is still growing and evolving, and hopefully one day they can have more solutions and ways to help their patients.

Chapter References

1. Gannotta, R., Malik, S., Chan, A. Y., Urgun, K., Hsu, F., & Vadera, S. (2018). Integrative Medicine as a Vital Component of Patient Care. *Cureus*, *10*(8), e3098. https://doi.org/10.7759/cureus.3098

2. Ee, C., Lake, J., Firth, J. *et al.* An integrative collaborative care model for people with mental illness and physical comorbidities. *Int J Ment Health Syst* **14,** 83 (2020). https://doi.org/10.1186/s13033-020-00410-6

3. Lake, J., M.D. (2007). INTEGRATIVE MENTAL HEALTH CARE: FROM THEORY TO PRACTICE, PART 1. *Alternative Therapies in Health and Medicine, 13*(6), 50-6.

4. Lake, J., Helgason, C., & Sarris, J. (2012). Integrative Mental Health (IMH): paradigm, research, and clinical practice. *Explore (New York, N.Y.), 8*(1), 50–57. https://doi.org/10.1016/j.explore.2011.10.001

Chapter 19.
Black Holistic Health Stress Model

BLACK HOLISTIC HEALTH OVERVIEW

Leading up to the release of this book I was able to host my first Black Health + Wellness Virtual Summit (2023). As a speaker for this event, I spoke on the topic of Black Holistic Health, and from this talk I decided to share the Black Holistic Health Stress Model.

So, for this model, **black holistic health** is comprised of seven distinct components. The first three are considered primary components and the remaining four are considered secondary components of black holistic health.

PRIMARY BLACK HOLISTIC HEALTH COMPONENTS

1. *Physical Health* : the overall health and function of the physical body and its systems.

2. *Mental Health* : emotional and psychological well-being of an individual. Including their ability to live a productive life and function in society.

3. *Spiritual Health* : connecting with God while loving and serving others. Includes spiritual practices (i.e., prayer, meditation, etc.).

SECONDARY BLACK HOLISTIC HEALTH COMPONENTS

4. *Financial Health* : our overall financial stability. Includes financial literacy, financial growth, savings, investments, retirement plans, etc.

5. *Social Health* : our meaningful relationships with relatives and nonrelatives. Includes the ability to build and maintain relationships with others. These relationships typically make up our support system.

6. *Environmental Health* : the state of one's environment. Includes housing, neighborhood, water, air, noise, etc. This definition has been further expanded to include higher crime rates, areas/housing with a lot of rodents and other pests, and lots of visible trash and abandoned properties in the neighborhood.

7. *Sexual Health* : This definition includes (+/-) sexually transmitted infections (STIs) along with the state of one's uncoerced sexual practices and sexuality.

BLACK HOLISTIC HEALTH STRESS MODEL

Now that the 7 components of Black Holistic Health have been introduced, we can now discuss the Black Holistic Health Stress Model. This model will attempt to illustrate how stress can impact the total holistic health of black people and how the seven individual components of black holistic health can impact each other.

Stress Response Of The Body

Our body responds when we are in various situations that are deemed "stressful," and a part of this response includes the release of epinephrine and cortisol. Epinephrine is both a neurotransmitter (helps neurons communicate) and a hormone. Cortisol is a steroid hormone that is released by the adrenal glands. Both epinephrine (also referred to as adrenaline) and cortisol (primary stress hormone) are important during the "fight or flight" response when your sympathetic nervous system has been activated. The body's response to stress is meant to be a temporary response in the body. However, chronic stress can keep the body in a fight or flight state longer than normal and this can lead to issues. Elevated epinephrine and cortisol levels over time can have a number of effects on one's holistic health.

When released Cortisol can:
- Increase blood glucose levels
- Increase blood pressure
- Raise heart rate

What Can Cause Stress?
(These are just examples; this is not an exhaustive list)
- Job/Supervisor
- Loss of employment/ Underemployed
- Low Wages/ Lack of Scheduled Working Hours
- Family Conflict
- Marriage/Romantic Relationship Issues
- Infidelity
- Children/Parenting
- School
- Bills and financial responsibilities
- Homelessness and Housing Instability
- Feeling unsafe in your community
- Inadequate Housing (run down housing)
- Living without utilities (no heat, running water etc.)
- Rodent and Pest Infestation
- Food Insecurity
- Illness
- Working excessively
- Environmental factors (dirty/unclean water, noise, air pollution etc.)
- Incarcerated loved ones or being incarcerated

- Transportation (i.e. impounded vehicle, repossessed vehicle, expensive car repairs, public transportation hard to access etc.)
- Low Income/Poverty/Financial Issues
- Racism and Discrimination
- Lack of support from family and friends
- Being a single parent with no help
- Death of a loved one (emphasis on tragic death such as a child being shot and killed)
- Divorce
- Infertility/Miscarriage/Still birth/Infant death
- Lack of funds for personal hygiene products, personal grooming, and washing clothing.
- Ongoing abuse and trauma (domestic violence etc.)
- Addiction

How Stress Impacts Black Holistic Health

Listed below are some ways that stress can impact **the three primary components of the Black Holistic Health Model** (physical health, mental health, and spiritual health).

Physical Health – Chronic stress can have a significant impact on physical health. The body's stress response is meant to be short term. When the body's stress alarm system stays on due to chronic stress it can increase one's risk of:

- Cardiovascular disease
- Hypertensions
- Type 2 Diabetes
- Issues with digestive system
- Muscle weakness or muscle pain
- Problems with sleep
- Weight gain
- Weakened immune system
- Headaches

- Osteoporosis
- Fatigue

Mental Health and Behavior – When our body's stress response stays activated it can also affect our mental health. Chronic stress can put an individual at risk for:
- Anxiety
- Depression
- Substance Abuse
- Issues with memory and staying focused
- Declining performance in school/work
- Isolation
- Difficulties building and maintaining healthy relationships.

Spiritual Health – Chronic stress can impact spiritual health.

- Stress can result in a decline in prayer, fasting, attending religious services, disconnecting from your faith community, and other practices.

- Faith, spirituality, and serving others could be removed as a priority due to stress taking a toll on an individual.

- Faith and belief system could be completely dismantled due to chronic stress connected to personal hardship and extreme trauma.

Listed below are some ways that stress can impact **the four secondary components of the Black Holistic Health Model** (financial health, social health, environmental health, and sexual health):

Social Health – It might not be an initial thought but over time stress can impact our social health and the relationships in our lives.
- Avoiding communication with others.

- Periods of isolation from friends, family, co-workers, or romantic partners.
- Struggles with maintaining healthy relationships.
- Frustration/outbursts directed towards others can result in the breakdown of relationships including marriage, which can increase isolation and frustration, and this can exacerbate other issues.
- Being estranged from children or extended family members is also a possibility.

Financial Health – When dealing with stress sometimes it can influence our financial health.
- Poor financial decisions and impulsivity with finances.
- Decrease in work performance (behavior) which can result in diminished job hours or termination of employment which can result in increased stress and further depreciated financial health.

Environmental Health – Stress over time can make an individual more susceptible to environmental toxins and pollutants. Furthermore, the recognition of environmental health issues can also be a source of stress (lead in water, noise pollution, manufacturing plant releasing toxins etc.)

Sexual Health – Stress can result in a decreased desire for sex which can impact romantic relationships. However, some people have an increased sex drive when stressed. Lastly, stress can be associated with non-consensual sexual events (sexual assault) or even contracting STIs from a partner.

HOW THE 7 BLACK HOLISTIC HEALTH COMPONENTS IMPACT EACH OTHER WHEN STRESS IS INVOLVED

Below is a text outline and chart to show a few ways stress disrupts Black Holistic Health. The text outline also gives descriptions of how various components of the Black Holistic

Health Model can impact each other. Up and down arrows refer to increase or decrease. A down arrow next to mental health would mean a decrease in one's overall mental health. An up arrow by financial health would indicate an increase in one's overall financial health, which is a good thing.

↑ STRESS

- Sleeping issues can exacerbate stress which can directly impact several components of your holistic health.

- Racism and discrimination are both sources of stress and/or they can exacerbate stress.

- Multiple factors (stressors) can result in a person dealing with chronic stress

- Stress can impact and disrupt holistic health as a whole

↓ PHYSICAL HEALTH

- The stress response of the body results in the release of epinephrine and Cortisol. Cortisol is considered the main stress hormone. Cortisol can increase the heart rate, blood pressure, and blood glucose levels. Overtime this can increase the risk for diabetes, atherosclerosis, kidney disease and cardiovascular disease.

- *If a diagnosis occurs* physical health issues can limit work and income (financial health). Also, costs associated with medication and care can be burdensome (stress). Insurance and financial issues can be a barrier to proper preventative care and monitoring and treating currently diagnosed health conditions.

- *Physical health issues can also lead to anxiety, depression, and isolation (i.e. terminal illness)*

↓ MENTAL HEALTH

- A decrease in mental health can result in declining performance in school and work including absenteeism. This can result in reduced work hours, suspension, or even termination can lead to a decrease in financial health can also lead to increased stress.

- Chronic stress can impact one's mental health and this could lead to declining performance at school which can lead to dismissal (college). School suspension can lead to unexpected financial obligations and school Financial aid can be restricted. This can be a financial burden and lead to increased stress.

- Mental health issues can limit work and income. Also, costs associated with medication and professional mental health services can be burdensome (stress). Insurance and finances can be a barrier to proper treatment for mental health concerns. This can cause people to have mental health concerns that go unmanaged, undiagnosed, or even untreated.

- Mental health issues can lead to isolation, diminished communication and the breakdown of relationships. (being ghosted by a parent, spouse filing for divorce, alienated from children, friendships ending abruptly etc.)

- Mental Health issues and general health issues can impact spiritual health due to a mental health diagnosis. This is especially true when there are faulty belief systems (i.e. mental illness means you do not pray enough).

- Research has shown that fasting is good for your physical and mental health including the reduction of stress. Furthermore, meditation and prayer are strongly believed to be beneficial to one's mental health.

↓ SPIRITUAL HEALTH

- Stress can impact spiritual health, and this can result in a decline in prayer, fasting, attending religious services, connecting with your faith community, and other practices.

- A lot of social ties can be directly connected to our faith and those in our faith community. When stress is present isolation and walking away from our faith community can occur and this could impact one's social health.

- Faith, spirituality, and serving others could be removed as a priority due to stress taking a toll on one's spiritual health
- Physical and mental health issues and diagnosis can lead to weakened or even abandoned faith.

↓ FINANCIAL HEALTH

- Individuals with lower income are more likely to live in neighborhoods where they have a greater chance of experiencing harm to their *environmental health* which can exacerbate stress.
- Finances play a huge role in a person's quality of life and can be a factor in chronic stress.
- Financial barriers can limit one's ability to get proper preventative health care and can completely hinder receiving adequate physical/mental health care.
- A lower income can mean living in a neighborhood with higher rates of crime. Lower income can also limit your ability to find housing in a neighborhood without negative environmental factors.
- Housing instability and food insecurity can also be associated with low financial health.
- Lastly there is research to suggest that a lower household income (poverty) make people more susceptible to multiple traumatic events which impacts one's holistic health and quality of life
- Financial issues can impact social health which could result in being estranged from family, losing business relationships, parenting and custody issues etc.

↓ ENVIRONMENTAL HEALTH

- Communities with higher levels of lead in water, paint, and soil. Lead can lead to a plethora of issues that affect physical health, mental health and behavior and can present barriers that hinder financial health
- Neighborhoods where pollutants (air, water etc.) are released by manufacturing companies

- Irritating noises including noise pollution

↓ SOCIAL HEALTH

- Social health can impact financial health. Going through a divorce can be costly. Custody battles and alienation from children can be problematic.
- The loss of business partnerships and social networking can also impact one's financial health.
- Family estrangement can also lead to a lack of support in a financial crisis.
- Physical or mental health issues can lead to isolation and distance from those that are normally the most important individuals in your life.
- In extreme cases an individual can be abandoned by those closest to them when an illness or disability (i.e. loss of mobility) is present.
- Struggles with relationships including marriage and child-parent relationships.
- Family turmoil (siblings, parents etc)

↓ SEXUAL HEALTH

- Social relationships, and personal beliefs including spiritual beliefs can play a role in one's sexual health.
- Some physical health issues can limit the ability to have free and healthy sexual relationships. (i.e. erectile dysfunction)
- Contracting STIs can impact physical health (i.e. discharge from genitals or anus, sores on/ near genitals or buttocks).
- A decrease in sexual health can affect a person's mental health.

On the next page there is a chart that is a visual of this text outline. The chart shows the 7 components of black holistic health, the way they can be impacted by stress and each other.

Chart 1. - Title: Black Holistic Health Stress Model Chart

Black Holistic Health Model - D'Andrea Bolden, MA

Free Arrows do not indicate direction instead they are used to indicate increase or decrease (down) of a Black Holistic Health Stress Model Component

I believe we have a "silent" lead crisis. We are seeing an increase of data and reports sharing that lead is in homes, soil, water, food, and other items. – D'Andrea Bolden

Other

Health Concerns

Chapter 20.
Black Children + Lead Exposure

I still remember when the announcements came out concerning the Flint, Michigan water crisis. I remember the news alerts and all the media coverage at that time. I recall thinking that it would not be a bad idea if all US residents that live in public housing and lower income neighborhoods test their water for lead. While writing this chapter there was an announcement about lead issues in Benton Harbor, Michigan. There was also a water crisis in Jackson, Mississippi that left residents with no running water for days. This is why I am a strong believer that everyone, especially those living in urban (black and brown) communities, should have their homes and water checked for lead.

What do we know about lead? Lead is a heavy metal that, even in small quantities, can cause serious health and behavioral problems, especially in children. Although a lot of efforts have been made to ensure that lead-based paint is removed from housing, the threat is still very real today. It is strongly believed that children living in housing built before 1978 and that live in housing below the federal poverty line have an increased risk of being exposed to lead.

The Dangers of Lead Exposure

Anything equivalent or above 5μg/dL (5 micrograms per deciliter) is considered elevated blood lead levels (BLL) in children. However, the CDC modified this to 3.5 μg/dL in 2022. In the US, the children with the highest BLL are African American children. Poverty and being black increase the likelihood of elevated BLL during childhood. It is believed that almost half of Americans have been exposed to lead.[1]

What happens when people are exposed to lead? Are you aware of the symptoms associated with elevated BLL? It is well documented that high lead levels in the blood can cause a plethora of issues. These issues can affect the health and behavior of the individuals impacted. Some research studies point towards a significant association between elevated blood lead levels and a decrease in cognition and intelligence (IQ scores), while other studies point towards an association of elevated BLL and some of the symptoms of ADHD. [1-8]

Individuals most at Risk of Lead Exposure[1-8]

1. Individuals that work at jobs that involve lead
2. Individuals living in housing built before 1978 that has not been renovated to remove lead-based paint
3. Children in low-income neighborhoods
4. Children under the age of six
5. Blacks in substandard housing
6. Living in a metropolitan area

Lead Exposure and Behavioral Symptoms[1-8]

- Aggression
- Antisocial Behavior
- Criminal Behavior
- Hyperactivity
- Impulsivity
- Delinquency

Lead Exposure and Physical Symptoms[1-8]

- Abdominal Pain
- Anemia
- Pica
- Seizures
- Hearing loss
- Speech issues
- Headaches
- Vomiting
- Hypertension
- Immunotoxicity
- Lower sperm count/abnormal sperm
- Coma
- Fatigue
- Loss of Appetite

Lead Exposure and Cognition[1-8]

- Reduced Attention Span/Distractibility
- Memory issues
- Lower IQ
- Lower Academic Performance
- Deficits in Executive Functioning
- Impulsivity
- Disorganization

Lead Exposure in Adults[1-9]

When examining elevated BLL in adults, there are associations with hypertension, mood disorders, miscarriage, stillbirth, or premature birth, pain in joints and muscles, headache, abdominal pain, sperm irregularities, and reduced sex drive. These symptoms are considered nonspecific which means that they do not point to a specific cause, and this helps explain why BLL can be overlooked or misdiagnosed. I was reading a study about lead exposure and criminology and the author hopes that courts will take elevated BLL into consideration and learn how it can cause neurological damage when sentencing defendants.[9] There are research studies that suggest lead exposure is linked to criminal behavior/incarceration and there are also studies that suggest this is not true.

Overall, it is important to understand that elevated BLL can affect both children and adults. However, children are more vulnerable to issues after being exposed to lead. It should be noted that in some cases the effects of childhood lead poisoning can last a lifetime. Damage to the nervous system (especially to the brain) and kidneys along with lowered intelligence and learning difficulties can impact a child's future all the way into adulthood.

Spread The Word

I saw a news article about a snack food product for children that was recalled due to elevated levels of lead in the snack. Lead exposure is a big deal, and we need to be more aware and spread the word. There are a lot of studies that have been shared publicly that address lead exposure, children, and the effects of elevated blood lead levels. However, I do not believe that most of the general public are aware of these studies. Every time I see another water crisis in an area with a lot of minorities in lower income communities, I wonder how many people instantly think about the water and environment where they currently reside.

We are seeing more lead exposure stories related to water in predominantly black and brown communities, and we cannot afford to ignore these issues. The damage that lead can cause to children and adults should be enough to cause an outcry. However, when people have no clue what lead is or the dangers that it poses, people just look at these instances and do not think much of it.

When you look at all the symptoms related to elevated BLL, it should make you think. How many of our black children are really impacted by elevated BLL, and could this be affecting their behavior and ability to thrive in school? How many black adults and children are experiencing symptoms of elevated BLL? Should black children be tested more often to ensure that they do not have elevated BLL or to identify it early and have it treated? This could be important because the damage caused by elevated BLL can be irreversible. This is a serious topic that needs to be addressed in every black home and predominantly black neighborhoods. This needs to be a topic in churches, schools, college campuses, barbershops/hair salons, and so on. People need to know what they are facing as it pertains to lead.

I believe we could potentially have a "silent" lead crisis on our hands. Lead is in homes, soil, water, food, and other items. Out of all the chapters in this book this one is the most important. I believe as black people we must become more aware of lead, where it can be found in our surroundings, and how it can potentially impact our health if we are exposed.

If you or someone you know has been exposed to lead, contact your healthcare provider, your public department of health, and your local/regional poison control center.

Chapter References

1. McFarland, M. J., Hauer, M. E., & Reuben, A. (2022). Half of US population exposed to adverse lead levels in early childhood. *Proceedings of the National Academy of Sciences, 119*(11). https://doi.org/10.1073/pnas.2118631119

2. Ramírez Ortega D, González Esquivel DF, Blanco Ayala T, Pineda B, Gómez Manzo S, Marcial Quino J, Carrillo Mora P, Pérez de la Cruz V. Cognitive Impairment Induced by Lead Exposure during Lifespan: Mechanisms of Lead Neurotoxicity. Toxics. 2021 Jan 28;9(2):23. doi: 10.3390/toxics9020023. PMID: 33525464; PMCID: PMC7912619.

3. Hou, S., Yuan, L., Jin, P. *et al.* A clinical study of the effects of lead poisoning on the intelligence and neurobehavioral abilities of children. *Theor Biol Med Model* 10, 13 (2013). https://doi.org/10.1186/1742-4682-10-13

4. Mayo Foundation for Medical Education and Research. (2022, January 21). *Lead poisoning*. Mayo Clinic. https://www.mayoclinic.org/diseases-conditions/lead-poisoning/symptoms-causes/syc-20354717

5. Schwaba, T., Bleidorn, W., Hopwood, C. J., Gebauer, J. E., Rentfrow, P. J., Potter, J., & Gosling, S. D. (2021). The impact of childhood lead exposure on adult personality: Evidence from the United States, Europe, and a large-scale natural experiment. *Proceedings of the National Academy of Sciences, 118*(29). https://doi.org/10.1073/pnas.2020104118

6. Bellinger DC. Childhood Lead Exposure and Adult Outcomes. *JAMA.* 2017;317(12):1219–1220. Doi:10.1001/jama.2017.1560

7. Mohammadyan, M., Moosazadeh, M., Borji, A., Khanjani, N., & Somayeh, R. M. (2019). Investigation of occupational exposure to

lead and its relation with blood lead levels in electrical solderers. *Environmental Monitoring and Assessment, 191*(3), 1-9. https://doi.org/10.1007/s10661-019-7258-x

8. Delgado CF, Ullery MA, Jordan M, Duclos C, Rajagopalan S, Scott K. Lead Exposure and Developmental Disabilities in Preschool-Aged Children. J Public Health Manag Pract. 2018 Mar/Apr;24(2):e10-e17. doi: 10.1097/PHH.0000000000000556. PMID: 28257404.

9. Kittilstad, E. (2018). REDUCED CULPABILITY WITHOUT REDUCED PUNISHMENT: A CASE FOR WHY LEAD POISONING SHOULD BE CONSIDERED A MITIGATING FACTOR IN CRIMINAL SENTENCING. *Journal of Criminal Law & Criminology, 108*(3), 569-595.

Chapter 21.
Black Women + Pregnancy

Pregnancy is an incredibly beautiful experience. The journey and process of bringing forth life is different for every woman and for each pregnancy. I wish I could say that I was one of the women blessed to have a storybook pregnancy. You know, like the pregnancy you see on TV where the woman wakes up, they vomit once, take a pregnancy test and nine months later they are smiling and holding a beautiful baby. There are some women that have very enjoyable pregnancies with few or no complications, but for many women that is not the case.

According to the CDC, up to twenty-six percent of all pregnancies end in miscarriage. [1] It was also shared that eighty percent of early pregnancy loss occurs during the first trimester.[1] Did you know that one in one hundred and sixty stillbirths occur annually, which is about 24,000 stillborn children every year?[2] What I found most interesting is that one of the risk factors that increases the chance of having a pregnancy ending with a stillbirth is being of the black race.[2] I was shocked when I read this but I also felt that this was very important and should be shared. I can only speak for myself when I say that after having two children, I was completely ignorant of all this information.

One thing that has been getting more attention is the number of black women that die from preventable complications related to childbirth and this is believed to be associated with infant death. It has been shared that blacks have the highest infant mortality rate in the United States. I can recall seeing some very publicized stories of black women dying during or shortly after giving birth. But like many other people, I never connected the dots or researched this matter to get a better understanding of this issue.

It is strongly believed that better care would have prevented the death of some black infants and mothers, especially when there are still racial disparities in modern healthcare.[3] Poverty can be an obvious factor with lower income women being more likely to forego maternal care, but even black women with higher incomes face these same issues. It has been stated that the pregnancy-related mortality ratio for black women over the age of thirty per 100,000 live births is four to five times higher than white women.[3] Overall, they shared that black women are two to three times more likely to die from pregnancy-related complications when compared to white women.

As a black woman that has gone through two bittersweet pregnancies, this was all very shocking for me. I say bittersweet because of the complications I endured amid being blessed with two beautiful children. Growing up I always knew that I wanted a big family, but after two traumatic pregnancies I realized that was not going to happen for me.

My personal pregnancy stories are disturbing when I share them with other people, but I wanted to share my experience in this chapter since I am a black mother that has gone through two pregnancies.

During my first pregnancy I was a single mother on Medicaid, and I share that because I do feel that having public government insurance played a role in my birth experience during my first pregnancy. During the first trimester I was told that I had placenta previa because the placenta was partially covering the opening of my cervix. I was then told that I needed to be on pelvic rest for several weeks. After that day, placenta previa was not mentioned at any prenatal appointment again until my third trimester.

Other than an aversion to certain smells and nausea to certain foods, my first pregnancy went smoothly until the beginning of the third trimester. I can recall at one doctor's visit when I was around seven months along, my doctor wanted to get an opinion from a second doctor; we will call them Dr. A, and Dr. B. When I had one of my scheduled appointments with Dr. A, he invited Dr. B in to give a second opinion about concerns over placenta previa as the baby was growing quickly, my uterus was expanding, and my due date was getting closer. Dr. B believed that due to the location of the placenta and other factors that there was a good chance as my uterus continued to expand with the pregnancy that the placenta could become detached completely from the wall of the uterus specifically during labor. However, my doctor, or Dr. A, disagreed and felt that everything would be fine and that we should move forward and disregard this second medical opinion.

A few weeks had passed since that appointment with Dr. A and Dr. B, and the holidays were quickly approaching. I had just completed a semester of classes. It was mid-December, and I could feel that I was beginning to slow down. Although my baby was not due until February, instinct kicked in and I finished the baby's room and packed my bag for the hospital.

On December 24th at around thirty-three or thirty-four weeks (about eight months), I woke up to use the bathroom and when I stood up, I felt a gush. My assumption at the time was that my water had broken, and that amniotic fluid was leaking down my legs. Immediately I rushed to the bathroom and within moments I heard a loud thud. I looked on the floor and saw what was eventually determined to be a gigantic blood clot. The thing was huge; it was the size of a T-bone steak. I was in shock and did not know what to do so I had some family members take me to the local hospital. When I arrived, the medical staff determined quickly that I was having contractions and going into premature labor. However, it was still too early for me to give birth since my due date was February 7th. The hospital staff administered a shot to stop the premature labor and shared that my local hospital would not be equipped to handle a premature baby if I were to deliver any time soon. I was admitted into the hospital and stayed for one night before they released me to go home.

Two days later I was back in the hospital for the exact same reason, but this time I was being kept for observation. The doctor I had been seeing for prenatal care during most of my pregnancy (Dr. A) was now on vacation for the holidays and he left another doctor in his place. But once I was hospitalized the second doctor was unavailable and on vacation too, leaving me with a third doctor that I had never met. The third doctor was a female, and she was also pregnant and looked to be around seven or eight months pregnant. This doctor made the decision to send me to a hospital in a larger city that was better equipped to provide care for me and if necessary, they could handle a premature baby if I were to deliver early.

So, on December 30th I was transported by ambulance to the new hospital, and I can admit that I was relieved. I was in a hospital that was better equipped to provide care for me and my unborn child. When I arrived, I was told that I would be staying in the hospital until my due date in February. This was not good news for me. If you have ever been in the hospital, you know how uncomfortable it is, and being pregnant made things tough. Although I was glad to be there, I was not looking forward to staying in the hospital for that long. I felt like I was counting down for my release date and not my due date.

Well, oddly enough, I did not even make it to one week before I went into labor. I woke up on January 3rd and the bed pad that was beneath me showed that I was hemorrhaging a little and that my water might have broken. I reached out to the nurse to let them know that something was going on. Once I shared this with the nurse, she informed the doctor who had me moved immediately to labor and delivery.

I can still remember being in labor for hours and I never dilated past three centimeters. I was shocked because on TV it all happens so quickly, but, of course, real life is so different. After a while I can recall very vividly the doctor saying that he was going to administer Pitocin which would intensify uterine contractions. I asked the doctor if that could cause further bleeding and issues especially with me dealing with placenta previa the entire pregnancy. I shared how this was not a good idea. He said that he saw no potential issues and ignored me. Black women really do get ignored and dismissed by those who are in the healthcare system.

After being administered Pitocin, everything went south very quickly. The contractions got strong, and the pain was getting unbearable. Except for when I had to the use the bathroom, I was constantly hooked up to monitors and machines. After a few hours I can remember lying on the bed when the nurses and doctors appeared suddenly. They looked at the monitors and I could tell by the looks on their faces that something was not right. Within a matter of a few moments, I was stuffed into a wheelchair and medical staff sprinted me down to the operating room. I was only told that my baby's heart rate had dropped and nothing more. Shortly thereafter, my daughter was delivered by emergency c-section just over five weeks early. Initially there was an assumption that she would need to go to NICU due to anticipated issues with breathing and feeding, but we were blessed that she had no complications; she was discharged with me.

Post-delivery I can still remember how I received very subpar care. I can still remember one of the nurses ripping my catheter out. I was left in a hospital room with the door closed and no one came to check on me. How could they be so cold and cruel after I had just had major surgery? One of the nurses took my baby out of the room and left me alone. I can still recall how I mustered up enough strength to go down and get my baby out of the nursery. Sadly, she was put in the nursery off to the side by herself away from the other babies. As I am reminiscing on the situation, I am shaking my head. I was very young at this time and did not know any better. Plus, I was in the hospital all alone - just me and my newborn baby girl.

It sounds like a happy conclusion should come next, right? Wrong; it was not until seven and a half years later when my husband and I were expecting our son that I was told that my first pregnancy was an emergency c-section due to placenta abruption. What?

Why didn't anyone tell me? I could not believe my ears. Placenta abruption means the placenta had completely detached from the inner wall of my uterus. This is very serious, and in some cases, it can result in stillbirth. I was shocked that my baby's life was in more danger than I knew and that I found out almost eight years later.

With my second pregnancy I was eight years older and married. Sadly, my second pregnancy was much worse than the first. I know you were hoping for some great news with my second pregnancy, but it was like eight and a half months of torture while being ignored by doctors. First, I had morning sickness until the very end of the pregnancy. Every morning my daughter or my husband would hand me a bucket to vomit in after I woke up. I would vomit at work, in the car, at home, or anywhere else. For months all I could eat was apples and cantaloupe; I could not hold anything else down. I would also suck on sunflower seeds and hot Cheetos because it would help to settle my stomach. Even if I felt that I could eat more, I would still throw up shortly afterwards.

When I was in the second trimester of this pregnancy, I can remember being unable to eat or drink for three days and the hospital gave me something for my throat because my throat was swollen and burning at this time. I can remember when I began coughing up blood and I was told by people to suck it up because that is a part of pregnancy. I have yet to find coughing up blood listed as a symptom of pregnancy.

Because of my age and the history associated with my first pregnancy, I was considered high-risk the second time around and I had to schedule double the number of doctor's visits than a woman with a normal pregnancy. Although I had a set of doctors that I saw, they would send me to high-risk pregnancy specialists for further evaluation. I can remember at most appointments I was told that my son might not make it. They also told me that due to his size, a vaginal birth was no longer an option and that I had to have a c-section again.

With this pregnancy I was diagnosed with gestational diabetes, and it took quite a while to meet with the dietitian and get the medication to get my blood glucose levels under control. I did not begin taking insulin until my seventh or eighth month of pregnancy. By that time, the high blood glucose had led to excess amniotic fluid which caused me to begin to measure at full term in the month of May, but I was not due until September. It was also the cause of my son being too large to deliver vaginally.

I can remember one day in July my blood sugar had spiked to over four hundred, and I had to be rushed out of my husband's mother's funeral to the hospital. This was an extremely low point for me, and it was beyond frustrating. The doctor initially sent me home very quickly, but then he called and told me to come back, and I was admitted to the hospital. I stayed for one night until they were able to get my blood sugar levels normal and under control.

The week prior to this incident I woke up one day and my legs and feet were so swollen that when I walked, I could see and feel fluid moving on the top of my feet. I could no longer wear shoes at that point because my feet were so big. My feet are naturally small and narrow. I was already having issues working because the excess amniotic fluid and the weight of the baby were pressing on my nerves, and I would have moments where I would struggle to walk because I could not move. So, when I asked my doctor if I could get a note to take maternity leave in July, she told me no because I was perfectly fine. Although I could no longer wear shoes and I struggled to walk, I was expected to keep working. I decided at that point to take my maternity leave anyway, and for weeks I could only get out of bed to use the bathroom. During this time, I was supposed to be at doctor appointments every single day of the week, but I had no strength to get out of bed at this point. The doctor's office would keep calling, but I had no strength to get to the appointments.

This lasted for another month until I delivered my son via an emergency c-section. After a long terrible eight months, I was at a stress test appointment, and they could not get my baby to move. They tried for hours and there was no movement whatsoever. They performed an ultrasound and there was no movement. At this point my blood pressure was measuring extremely high and I was swollen and barely able to get around anymore. It was decided at this point that I should be admitted into the hospital again.

That night, after what felt like eternity, my son was delivered via emergency c-section. Can you believe that the doctor told my husband he did not believe that both me and my son would survive? My husband was asked who he wanted to save - me or my baby boy. Thank God we both survived because God surely had a plan. So, when my son was born, he was almost eleven pounds, and the medical staff checked him thoroughly to ensure that he did not have issues from gestational diabetes. Everything checked out and he was fine.

After a few days everything seemed okay, and we were released to go home two days later. The day after we went home, my body went haywire. I kept going from extremely hot to extremely cold. I would go from shivering to sweating within a matter of minutes. My son was born towards the end of the month of August, so it was hot outside. I was turning the furnace on because I was shivering and then after a few minutes I would switch the air conditioner on because I was so hot. I could not figure out what was going on and I tried to lay down, but I knew something was not right, so my husband took me and my 3-day old baby back to the hospital. By the time we got there I was screaming in pain. After my vitals were checked it was determined that my blood pressure was elevated. In fact, my blood pressure was considered 'stroke level' and the medicine that they administered via IV could not get it down. The doctor in charge then ordered tests and he ordered an ultrasound believing that something was left in my womb from the c-section, but nothing was found.

For hours they gave me pain medicine and blood pressure medicine, and nothing was working. The doctor said I had all the signs of an infection, but they could not figure out where the infection was located, and my blood pressure was not budging. So, I sat miserably in ER being pumped with medicine for hours until the pain began to lessen, and my blood pressure started to go down.

I was in so much pain after the c-section that it was hard for me to walk. Getting to the bathroom in our small two-bedroom apartment was a dreaded task. You know how women go for a follow up visit after having a baby? When I went to my follow-up appointment the week after the birth of my son I stood on the scale, and I had lost over fifty pounds. My skin was hanging, and I looked like an elderly woman, and I was not even thirty years old.

My body was tired from a pregnancy where I was throwing up every day until the pregnancy was over. I was swollen, I had gestational diabetes, my blood pressure was elevated, and I could barely eat throughout the duration of the pregnancy.

What stings the most is that when I have discussions with white women about pregnancy they are treated with a much higher regard. The doctors are more proactive versus in my case they were always reactive. There seems to be a lack of compassion for black mothers. After two pregnancies, one while on government insurance and the other with private insurance, the only difference I saw was slightly better treatment in the hospital after birth when I was on private insurance.

I know that my story is personal, but I also know as a black woman that my story is common. I can remember reading about how Serena Williams had to demand proper treatment when experiencing symptoms that were related to a serious health issue after delivering her first baby. That cause me to believe that money and fame will not protect you from being ignored or dismissed as a black woman receiving care.

At this point I do not believe that we (black women) get equal care and compassion as other mothers. Also, I do not believe that we are taken seriously or given the same level of respect as non-black mothers. It is important that black mothers understand how to advocate for themselves. It is important to have safe spaces for these discussions. Lastly, it is imperative that more black physicians, nurses, midwives, and other black professionals are available to provide services to pregnant black mothers and newborn babies because representation matters.

Chapter References

1. Dugas C, Slane VH. Miscarriage. [Updated 2021 Jun 29]. In: StatPearls [Internet]. Treasure Island (FL): StatPearls Publishing; 2021 Jan-. Available from: https://www.ncbi.nlm.nih.gov/books/NBK532992/

2. Centers for Disease Control and Prevention. (2020, November 16). *What is stillbirth?* Centers for Disease Control and Prevention. Retrieved from https://www.cdc.gov/ncbddd/stillbirth/facts.html.

3. Centers for Disease Control and Prevention. (2019, September 6). *Racial and ethnic disparities continue in pregnancy-related deaths*. Centers for Disease Control and Prevention. https://www.cdc.gov/media/releases/2019/p0905-racial-ethnic-disparities-pregnancy-deaths.html.

Chapter 22.
Black Women + Fibroids

I can honestly say that over the years I have lost count of the wives, mothers, sisters, and friends that were diagnosed with fibroids. The number of women that I know who are facing fertility issues, having hysterectomies, or other surgical procedures because of fibroids is astounding.

Originally, this topic was not going to be a part of this book until I saw something that caught my attention online. I was reading an article which triggered me to begin researching more information about black women and fibroids.

Although it was common to hear black women talking about fibroids, initially, I did not put much thought into this topic. However, over time I can say that in the back of my mind I was wondering why this was happening so much to black women. Was it genetic? Is diet a factor? Either way I became extremely interested and started looking for answers.

First, I wanted to understand fibroids. A fibroid is a benign or non-cancerous growth located outside or inside of a woman's uterus. According to the Mayo Clinic, fibroids happen during a woman's childbearing years and a lot of women have fibroids and do not know it because they do not experience any symptoms.[1] Those that do experience symptoms typically attest to several of the symptoms listed below.

- Heavy menstrual bleeding

- Menstrual periods lasting more than a week
- Pelvic pressure or pain
- Frequent urination
- Difficulty emptying the bladder
- Constipation
- Backache or leg pains

Have you ever wondered what is causing the growth of these fibroids? I pondered this question as I started to research this topic. The Mayo Clinic shared four factors that, based on research studies, seem to be associated with fibroid growth. The four factors are genetic changes, hormones, other growth factors (ex: insulin-like growth factor), and extracellular matrix.[1] The Mayo Clinic also shared that estrogen and progesterone hormones that affect the uterine lining during the menstrual cycle, can play a role in the actual growth of fibroids.[1]

It is believed that upwards of 80% of black women will have fibroids by the age of fifty.[2] This number is not exact because all women with fibroids do not experience symptoms and women are not always screened for fibroids. This means that the number of women that experience fibroids could be higher.

It is strongly believed that being of African ancestry is considered a significant risk factor for fibroids.[2] Did you know that fibroids in African American women are bigger and grow faster than other groups of women? Did you know that African American women are more likely to have surgery for fibroids than any other group of women? Although fibroids impact African American women disproportionately, it is not fully understood why. It has been shared that diet, abuse, and vitamin D deficiency are factors that increase the risk of fibroids.[2]

In the United States, fibroids are the most prevalent reason for hysterectomies. Outside of a hysterectomy there are several other options to treat fibroids including medical therapies, surgery, uterine artery embolization, and oral contraceptives.[2-3] I was so relieved to see that not only is there more research to help us understand fibroids and black women, but there are also organizations that are dedicated to the uterine health of black women.

News Flash! Before I could finish authoring this book there was a recent buzz in the news about a link between hair relaxers and uterine cancer. It makes me ponder if there is also an association between hair relaxers and fibroids in black women. Research needs to be conducted and conversations need to be had.

Chapter References

1. https://www.mayoclinic.org/diseases-conditions/uterine-fibroids/symptoms-causes/syc-20354288

2. Eltoukhi, H. M., Modi, M. N., Weston, M., Armstrong, A. Y., & Stewart, E. A. (2014). The health disparities of uterine fibroid tumors for African American women: a public health issue. *American journal of obstetrics and gynecology, 210*(3), 194–199. https://doi.org/10.1016/j.ajog.2013.08.008

3. Zimmermann, A., Bernuit, D., Gerlinger, C., Schaefers, M., & Geppert, K. (2012). Prevalence, symptoms and management of uterine fibroids: an international internet-based survey of 21,746 women. *BMC women's health, 12*, 6. https://doi.org/10.1186/1472-6874-12-6

Chapter 23.
Arthritis

Arthritis is a disease that causes inflammation in joints. It can cause pain and stiffness for individuals diagnosed with arthritis. It is believed that arthritis can be inherited genetically, or it can be caused by immune system issues. As a young girl, I recall seeing older black women that suffered from arthritis, especially with their hands. I can remember looking at their hands and thought that it looked painful. I could see bones, and the skin on their hands was very tight.

I learned that most times arthritis can begin in the fingers and toes and that there are several types of arthritis. Listed below are five of the more well-known forms of arthritis.

1. Osteoarthritis (The most common form of arthritis and is found a lot in the hands, hips, and knees.)
2. Rheumatoid Arthritis (Autoimmune disease where the immune system attacks its own tissues, joints and can also attack internal organs. It can cause inflammation that leads to bone erosion and deformities of the joints.)
3. Gout (Painful form of arthritis that tends to affect the big toe.)
4. Ankylosing spondylitis (Affects the joints and ligaments of the spine.)
5. Childhood Arthritis (Arthritis in children.)

It makes sense now, but I never realized that gout was a form of arthritis. I can still remember my grandfather having gout and how he would be upset and crying from having flareups. However, these flareups were caused by what he was eating and drinking while ignoring the advice from his doctors.

It is widely accepted that arthritis is a progressive condition that can worsen over time. Out of all the types of arthritis, rheumatoid arthritis is considered the most unpredictable and has the most complications.

Rheumatoid Arthritis is most common in women and typically develops between the ages of thirty and sixty.[1]

Risk Factors for Arthritis

1. Age
2. Gender
3. Overweight/Obese
4. Injuries
5. Muscle Weakness
6. Family History

Arthritis is a critical concern for the aging black population in the United States. It is estimated that just over twenty-two percent of American adults with arthritis are black. Some researchers have shared that older blacks have severe arthritic joint pain that impacts mobility and decreases daily functions.[2] Other research has suggested that black patients with arthritis are less likely to have treatment or corrective surgery to address their pain.

As with many other health issues, blacks with arthritis are more prone to not getting adequate care and having more severe symptoms.[2] Racial disparities are common and have a major impact on the health of black people, including those with arthritis.

Chapter References

1. *Rheumatoid arthritis - orthoinfo - AAOS*. OrthoInfo. (n.d.). https://orthoinfo.aaos.org/en/diseases--conditions/rheumatoid-arthritis/

2. Booker SQ, Tripp-Reimer T, Herr KA. "Bearing the Pain": The Experience of Aging African Americans With Osteoarthritis Pain. Glob Qual Nurs Res. 2020 Jun 3;7:2333393620925793. doi: 10.1177/2333393620925793. PMID: 32548212; PMCID: PMC7271276.

Chapter 24.

Black Men + Prostate Cancer

What is prostate cancer? Why is prostate cancer a big concern for black men? What do we know about black men and prostate cancer?

First, what is the prostate? The prostate is a gland found in the male reproductive system underneath the bladder. Prostate cancer is only relevant to men because women do not have a prostate.

Prostate cancer is the overgrowth of cells in the prostate (gland) of biological males. According to data, black males have a greater risk for developing prostate cancer than any other group (4.2%). Furthermore, prostate cancer has been found to be more aggressive and have a different genetic profile in black males. The incidence rate and mortality rate for prostate cancer is believed to be highest in black American males.[1]

- Black males are twice as likely to develop prostate cancer, and more than two times as likely to die from it.[2]

Symptoms of Prostate Cancer

- Difficulties urinating
- Decreased force in the stream of urine
- Blood in the urine
- Blood in the semen
- Bone pain

- Weight loss (unexplained/unintentional)
- Erectile dysfunction

Risk Factors for Prostate Cancer

1. Age
2. Family History
3. Being a black male

Black males tend to have a worse outcome because they are less likely to be screened and receive treatment for prostate cancer. Some researchers have considered whether black males need to be screened for prostate cancer at a younger age than other groups because black American males have the highest rates for prostate cancer in the world.[1]

Prostate screening recommendations by age have been released by the U.S. Preventive Services Task Force (USPSTF). The USPSTF is an independent group of experts that specialize in preventative medicine. Not everyone agrees with their recommendation for prostate screening.

Experts have shared that in some cases the growth rate is slow and that sometimes men will die of other causes before prostate cancer becomes advanced.[2] Also, it is suggested that men under forty and men over seventy do not need to undergo prostate cancer screening.

It is important for black males to have a PCP (primary care physician) and get all the necessary tests and screenings that are recommended for preventative care.

Chapter References

1. Hinata, N., & Fujisawa, M. (2022). Racial Differences in Prostate Cancer Characteristics and Cancer-Specific Mortality: An Overview. *The world journal of men's health*, 40(2), 217–227. https://doi.org/10.5534/wjmh.210070

2. Worthington, J. F. (n.d.). *Prostate Cancer and African Ancestry.* Prostate Cancer Foundation. https://www.pcf.org/c/prostate-cancer-and-african-ancestry/

Chapter 25.

Dental Care

It has bothered and shocked me how many black people grew up without going to the dentist. I had no clue that many black children did not have regular dental visits and cleanings. Sadly, many were never taught good oral hygiene either. When I refer to good oral hygiene practices, this includes brushing, flossing, recommended rinses, proper dental care, and professional care and maintenance.

Some things might seem basic or common sense, but not everyone is taught the importance of taking care of their teeth and going to the dentist on a regular basis. Some people do not understand that small children need to brush their teeth or the need to change their toothbrush on a regular basis. Some schools have toothbrushes and toothpaste in the classrooms because the children do not have these items readily available at home.

Based on published research, it is strongly believed that a considerable number of black children (lower income) do not have good oral health. This lack of good oral health includes untreated dental issues. In fact, the weight of poverty and healthcare disparities tends to have black households focus on health emergencies and not on preventative care.[1] What this means is that many black households, for several reasons, are more likely to seek healthcare/dental care only in an emergency and not regular checkups or routine appointments.

There are several reasons why this could happen, including the lack of transportation, lack of dental insurance, overcrowded clinics, or sometimes not understanding the importance of dental care.

It is estimated that over sixty percent of black dentists participate in Medicaid, however communities of color and black Americans who are sixty-five and older are more prone to not receiving dental health care.

Overall, a person's teeth and the state of their oral health can affect their confidence and self-esteem overall. We do not get to choose how our adult teeth look regarding imperfections, but we are able to control our level of personal care for our teeth. Sadly, I have seen a lot of adults in extreme pain due to a lot of tooth decay, but they were unable to get treatment because they were uninsured. I have seen clinics provide tooth extractions and other necessary services once or twice in a calendar year for low-income patients.

Our oral health impacts our overall health. Gum disease has been associated with diabetes, heart disease and other health issues. This is something I was unaware of for an exceptionally long time, but more people need to understand the importance of good oral health.

Chapter References

1. Assari, S., & Hani, N. (2018). Household Income and Children's Unmet Dental Care Need; Blacks' Diminished Return. *Dentistry journal, 6*(2), 17. https://doi.org/10.3390/dj6020017

Chapter 26.
The Impact of Poverty

"The rich man's wealth is his strong city: the destruction of the poor is their poverty." (Proverbs 10:15, KJV)

Poverty can be linked to almost every chapter and every section of this book. In real life, poverty has a way of affecting every aspect of a person's life. Poverty is a common fact that must be removed from the black population. Yes, there is poverty seen in every demographic, but too many black people are still bound by the chains of poverty. Let us take a moment and acknowledge that systemic racism, intentional barriers, family dysfunction, addiction, lack of good education, incarceration, and other factors have left many families in multi-generational poverty.

Working with people in poverty in the community for many years has taught me a lot. Number one - as black people we should not judge our brothers and sisters that are caught in cycles of poverty. Let us not frown upon our own people and silently agree with the same lies being perpetuated that if they wanted more out of life they would work hard, or they are "poor" because they are lazy. Those statements are nothing but lies, especially when a lot of low-income households have adults that work multiple jobs. We should always try to encourage and educate, even when it seems like our efforts and the resulting impact are worlds apart.

Our people need our love, help and support, not our criticism or looking down our noses at them like non-black people do. We should never cause financial harm to our own people for personal monetary benefits. This is important because on a global level, black people are heavily exploited by all others for financial gain.

When we look at the lives of others it is easy to see flaws, problems, and mistakes. Many people might not have made what would be deemed as the best choices in life, but they did the best they could with the hand that they were dealt. If you have never been in the grips of poverty, you might not understand the lives of those who have been in such a predicament.

Poverty is one of the most powerful forces that is crushing black people around the world. Where there is great poverty, there is a lot of hopelessness, trauma, mental illness, violence, crime, chaos, dysfunctional families, illiteracy, extreme substance abuse and neglected children. I hate poverty and what it does to the minds of black people. It is challenging to try and change the mindset of individuals that have been living in poverty. Poverty comes with so many challenges, and it seems like the needs and the crises never end.

In the US almost twenty percent of black Americans live below the federal poverty line. When looking at all impoverished households in the US, it is believed that twenty-two percent of all US households in poverty are black.

How Poverty Impacts Everyday Life

Diet

Many low-income neighborhoods are food deserts. This means that most people often do not have easy access to healthy food options and are surrounded by processed foods and fast foods which are not good for our health. The lack of a healthy diet can be a significant contributing factor to several diseases as mentioned in the first chapter of this book.

Employment

Poverty can also impact job opportunities because location, skill set, education, and credit can impact employment opportunities. Also, better-paying jobs are usually not in low-income neighborhoods, which means that transportation can be a barrier. The further away a job is from home, the more costs are involved in getting to work, and it can also mean a longer and more complicated commute. Longer commutes can affect the ability to parent their children, and it increases the need for daycare and other support. So, this means getting or keeping a better paying job is not always as easy as it seems.

Healthcare

High-end medical and mental health facilities are not typically located in low-income areas. Oftentimes the health clinics that are available in low-income areas do not have the same resources or quality of care as seen in more affluent neighborhoods. Quite often in lower-income communities, the medical staff will have many patients with limited time, so they must move quickly from one appointment to the next without a lot of patient interaction or time to address prominent issues.

Education

It has become more common for schools in low-income communities to be riddled with problems and have low performance and high dropout rates. Many children from low-income households rely on school meals due to food insecurity at home. Many educators have seen up close the number of children that lack the basic necessities and support to perform well at school.

Black children are brilliant, but many times their brilliance, creativity, and innovativeness are not seen because of poverty. Children go to school hungry, wearing dirty clothes, and need proper hair grooming. It can be a struggle for children to concentrate and perform well in school under those types of conditions.

Nationally, black children are shown to score lower consistently on all standardized testing and in core subjects when compared to their peers. [Please know that I am not an advocate for standardized testing.] It has been shared that 5.9 % of (US born) black individuals between ages sixteen and twenty-four are high school dropouts (not in school and have not earned a high school diploma or GED), and it is estimated that twenty-three percent of black adults have low literacy skills.[2-3]

Family Dynamics

Close to seventy percent of black children are raised in single parent homes primarily by their mothers. Unfortunately, some of these single mothers are fighting to stay above water, and many have little to no help. With these scenarios, some of our black children are being raised in poverty.

As a woman that was a single mother, I applaud and tip off my hat to those that are trying to make it happen. A lot of single mothers are doing their best. They should be applauded for their efforts as they try to hold on and keep moving forward. I acknowledge and understand the struggle of single mothers because I can relate to their experience. Those were some of the most exhausting and frustrating days of my life. I can remember feeling drained because when it is just you, there is no break - no days off - and you must keep going. I can also recognize now the toll it took on my body from working so hard and for so many hours. I can look back and see how my attitude and perspective on life changed under the constant stress and pressure of being a single parent.

Sadly, this non-stop pressure can lead to stress, anxiety, depression, and other health issues. Over the years we have all seen quite a few news headlines of single mothers having meltdowns or leaving their children somewhere and driving away. In a perfect world, children would be born to two parents that are ready and willing to care for them, but we know that this is not always the case for a lot of reasons.

The number of black children that do not have active fathers is saddening. (This is not referring to fathers that want to be active but are blocked intentionally by the efforts of the mother.) It is important to note that when fathers are absent, in many cases it causes the mother to be absent too because with no help, some single mothers are working 2-3 jobs. This sad reality means that if the father is not active, and the mother is always working, the children are missing quality time, teaching, training, guidance, and preparation for their future. It also leaves them vulnerable to abuse, gangs, and neglect. They can also have a lack of necessary structure, go without proper meals, and go without academic and daily support. Daily support includes healthy interactions with their parents.

So, when you consider overworked mothers that are stressed and tired and when there is also an absent father, we can see how school performance is not where it should be or why some kids are going to school with dirty clothes, hungry, and acting out in class.

The workload of single mothers can be a lot, so simple things like having the time to take their children to regular appointments and checkups can be difficult due to time constraints, work, or transportation issues.

These are some simple reasons that can help paint a picture on how generations can be stuck in poverty. If children are not being nurtured and prepared for adulthood in many cases, they can fail to thrive and remain trapped in poverty. Although many of these things can occur for other reasons, it is important to recognize how family dynamics are interconnected with poverty which can impact our health in some way, shape, or form.

Trauma

Poverty and all that comes with it can be very traumatic. In fact, it is believed that people who live in poverty are more prone to experience multiple traumatic events. So, it should not come as a shock that children that live in low-income households are more likely to have a higher adverse childhood experience (ACE) score.

Poverty has a way of impacting a person's entire life which makes it so hard to overcome this situation. However, there are several credible black voices that are committed to teaching, coaching, and educating our people to help them break free from poverty and live a more abundant life. The fight to get out of poverty is very hard but with a plan and consistency it is possible.

Chapter References

1. Fusco RA, Yuan Y, Lee H, Newhill CE. Trauma, Sleep and Mental Health Problems in Low-Income Young Adults. Int J Environ Res Public Health. 2021 Jan 28;18(3):1145. Doi: 10.3390/ijerph18031145. PMID: 33525425; PMCID: PMC7908203.

2. Parker, A., & ParkerHey, A. (2023, September 30). *US literacy rate statistics for 2023 (Trends & Data)*. Prosperity For All. https://www.prosperityforamerica.org/literacy-statistics/

3. National Center for Education Statistics. (2023). Status Dropout Rates. *Condition of Education*. U.S. Department of Education, Institute of Education Sciences.

Chapter 27.
Black Women + Hair Care

As a black woman I can say confidently that hair is incredibly significant for us. In fact, the hair care industry geared towards black women brings in over one trillion dollars annually. I would love to see more black entrepreneurs reap the benefits of this multi-trillion-dollar industry. Everybody is making money because of us, but that is another topic. Black women are the only women on the planet with such a unique texture of hair. Even other groups of people with darker or melanated skin still tend to have straight hair or hair that is not kinky, wooly, and as tightly coiled as ours.

Our hair is truly diverse and incredibly beautiful. However, over the years I have noticed that a lot of black women and younger black girls are struggling with chronic hair loss, breakage, shedding, and other issues.

My generation is hopefully the last of those that were forced to sit still as the hot comb nearly burned off our neck, face, and skin. I still have not-so-fond memories of getting my hair pressed straight. Many of us were traumatized by being told that we were "tender-headed" when in some instances the real problem was that someone was using way too much force on our hair. It was necessary for many my age or older to have our hair relaxed so that it was not "nappy" and much easier to comb and manage.

I can only speak for myself that wearing pressed, processed (Jheri curl), and chemically relaxed (straightened) hair was so common that natural hair was frowned upon when I was growing up and the comments were extremely negative. Thankfully, natural hair is now more accepted, and even celebrated by many black women.

Once I got older, I decided to go natural, but I had no clue how to care for my natural hair. Most of us were not taught how to care for our natural hair. There was so much to figure out and so much to learn. What products work best? What routine worked the best for hair care? How do you retain length? How do you deal with a head full of thick natural hair on a regular basis? These were all things that many of us have had to discover over time by trial and error.

I want to make it clear that I love all my black sisters whether relaxed, natural, bald, braided, locs, extensions or however you choose to wear your hair. This chapter is not about disagreeing on what is best for black hair but instead we are examining some of the hair-related health issues that are seen commonly with black women.

Okay, let us continue this discussion on hair.

Whenever you get your hair done, it typically gives you a boost of confidence and you feel your best. Nobody likes bad hair days, and nobody wants their hair to look a "mess," so to speak.

Historically, when we look back at our ancestors, many of them were made to feel negatively about their hair. It was called "nappy," ugly, dirty, and many other derogatory terms. In some places black women were forced to cover their hair in public.

Black hair, and black bodies, for that matter, were seen as a point of shame.

So, for me it is a breath of fresh air to see so many black women embracing their hair and wearing it with pride. Since we are always trendsetters and we are willing to pay for our hair care, many nonblack-owned companies are scrambling to create products that cater to our hair - whether it is relaxed, natural, braided, and so on. That is a topic for another discussion.

I wanted to understand why so many black women, especially younger women, were losing their hair. Growing up it seemed like most black women had a head full of hair, even if they decided to wear extensions or wigs. However, I have discovered that there are a lot of reasons why black women are losing their hair and some of the reasons are avoidable while others are not.

Alopecia

Black women love, love, love their hair. That said, alopecia can be an extremely sensitive and difficult topic to address. I personally know quite a few women that are either completely bald or close to being completely bald due to alopecia. I know that this cannot be easy for them. Shout out to the women that rock their bald heads with confidence; they deserve much respect.

Alopecia is the absence or partial loss of hair in areas where it would normally grow. There are several distinct types of alopecia.

- Alopecia aerta (patchy baldness) and female pattern hair loss are both genetic. Because they are genetic, the ability to prevent them is impossible. Alopecia aerta is an autoimmune disorder where your immune system attacks your hair follicles resulting in hair loss on the scalp and other parts of the body. The hair can grow back eventually, but it can fall out again.

- Alopecia totalis is a type of alopecia aerta that results in a completely bald head.

- Cicatricial alopecia is a permanent form of alopecia that is caused by inflammation at the hair follicles which destroys them. These follicles are then replaced by scar tissue which is what causes the hair loss to be permanent.

There is one form of alopecia that is completely preventable and that is traction alopecia. Traction alopecia is caused by excessive tension from braids, locs, and hair extensions. How many times have you seen braids pulled so tight there were bumps at the root of the hair, the scalp appeared to be painfully red, or you could see that the weight of the hair extensions was too much for the hair roots? Traction alopecia is happening to black women and girls at an alarming rate. I have seen so many women lose their hair due to traction alopecia, and it is frightening. Many times, not only did they miss the opportunity to go to a dermatologist, but they kept going to the same stylist, and continued to get hairstyles that would cause more damage. They did not see the need to care for their hair or let it rest and recover.

Traction alopecia is not genetic, and sometimes it can be prevented by going to a licensed professional hairstylist. I understand that some ladies are on a budget, but always try and find a professional to avoid unnecessary hair loss.

I have spoken with multiple licensed cosmetologists that have told me some of the horror stories that they have seen. People would come in with bald spots all over their head because a hair style was too tight or the extensions were too heavy when the individual had fragile hair already.

Sadly, by the time some of the women I know had finally realized that they had a form of alopecia, the damage had been done and it was far too late. If the hair is harmed continuously, the hair follicles can be damaged, and the hair loss can then become permanent.

Conditions that Cause Hair Loss

Although cosmetologists learn about a plethora of scalp and hair conditions, some things might require a trip to a dermatologist to get things under control. I have seen people go to the dermatologist because their entire scalp was inflamed, and their hair was falling out by the handfuls because they were allergic to something that was used on their hair.

I know for me, after I installed locs in my hair years ago and took the locs down, I was not able to wear extensions. I have tried because I used to wear hair extensions and wigs for years. But after removing the locs, my scalp was extremely sensitive to hair extensions and to a lot of hair products. So, I have had to adjust and find hairstyles and products that do not irritate my scalp. With my experience I found that getting braids became a burden as my scalp would burn and itch for days at a time. Eventually I found a way to be able to get my hair braided again. However, to avoid serious hair loss I realized that I had to make some substantial changes on the hair styles I chose and on the products that I used on my hair and scalp. Had I continued to do the same things, I could have had some irreversible issues with my hair and scalp.

Growing up in the 80s it was Jheri curls, press and curls, or relaxers. Most of the black women I grew up around were not taught about hair care, scalp care and things of that nature. We found out by trial and error, like we did for many other things.

Like everything else mentioned in this book, scalp issues and hair loss are nothing new to the black community. It was important that in this chapter I shared a list of some of the most common scalp conditions found amongst black people, especially women.

- Trichorrhexis nodosa (hair breakage due to weak points)
- Traction Alopecia (caused by hairstyling and can be avoided)
- Frontal Fibrosing Alopecia (regressive hairline, loss of hair on eyebrows and extremities)
- Scarring Alopecia (inflammatory condition that results in permanent hair loss)
- Allergic contact (due to contact with an irritant such as a product that is put on the scalp)
- Central Centrifugal Cicatricial Alopecia (causes permanent hair loss)
- Seborrheic Dermatitis (This is a chronic form of eczema)

Acknowledging Hair Loss

Hair loss can occur, as mentioned before, due to alopecia and from certain hairstyles, genetics, inflammation, scalp conditions, chemicals, or stress. Yes, stress can be associated with hair loss. I have seen women in tears because every time they touched their hair it was falling out. These same individuals went to the doctor and the source was deemed to be stress. After they got their stress levels under control, their hair stopped falling out.

Hair loss can be an overly sensitive, frustrating, and embarrassing talking point. Hair is significant for a lot of black women and the uncontrollable loss of hair can be a source of pain. For some women, hair loss also affects their self-confidence. No matter what the cause, hair loss can be a hard reality for some women to handle. I have seen some women shave it all off and rock a bald head with style and grace, but that is not the case for everyone. Losing your hair can be extremely traumatic and might require you to seek professional mental health counseling to help you cope.

If you or someone you know is suffering from hair loss, seek a professional that can pinpoint the cause. All hair loss is not permanent, and in some cases the hair can grow back. Also, find a licensed professional that has the knowledge and skill to care for your hair to avoid causing more damage to your scalp and hair follicles that could lead to permanent hair loss.

Chapter 28.
Sexual Health

I strongly believe that sexual health should not be completely disregarded when looking at black health holistically. Sex can impact a person's physical health (for example, pregnancy, STIs), mental health, finances (in terms of medicine, child support), and so on.

Having sex can increase your risk of contracting an STI (or sexually transmitted infection). It is imperative that you take the proper precautions and measures to ensure that you are safe. As society becomes more liberal towards sex, sexuality, and sexual experiences, some may experience some unwanted situations. Having sexual encounters with multiple partners while unprotected can have grave consequences. No one wants to be told that they have contracted HIV/AIDS, and there is no way to look at someone and know whether they are free from any type of transmittable disease.

Anyone who is sexually active needs to take the proper precautions and get regular checkups to ensure that they have not contracted an STI. It is equally important that your sexual partner(s) take(s) the same precautions to reduce the chance of infection.

Safe sex not only reduces the chance of contracting an STI; it also reduces the chance of pregnancies occurring. No pregnancy prevention method is one hundred percent foolproof, which is why I say that it reduces the chance of pregnancy, because it does not eliminate the possibility.

Sex also requires mutual respect and agreement between consenting adults. Participants should understand the importance of consent, boundaries and respecting the other parties that you are engaging with sexually.

I want to share some statistics relevant to black sexual health.

- As of 2018 it was reported by the CDC that over forty percent of new HIV cases were black people with over thirty percent identifying as black males. Furthermore, black males that identify as gay and bisexual accounted for over twenty-five percent of new HIV cases.[1]

- It was also shared that over forty percent of individuals diagnosed with HIV that passed away were black. It was noted that their actual death could have been other causes, but they were in the demographic of individuals living with HIV when they passed away.[1]

- Another source reported that almost sixty percent of new HIV cases among women were black women.[2]

- Nearly thirty-five percent of new Syphilis cases were reported among black people.[1]

- The number of black people diagnosed with gonorrhea was estimated to be almost eight times higher when compared to gonorrhea in individuals categorized as white.[1]

- Although contested, the CDC stood behind a 2010 report that stated nearly fifty percent of new herpes cases were diagnosed in black women.

- STIs can be associated with several symptoms. Although every STI is not the same, I created a brief list of symptoms that can occur.

  - Discharge from the penis
  - White, green, or yellow vaginal discharge
  - Testicles swollen or in pain (men)
  - Pain when urinating
  - Foul vaginal odor
  - Pain during intercourse (women)
  - Anal itching
  - Swollen lymph glands
  - Rash
  - Blisters or open sores (genital area, anal area, or area close by)
  - Fever

Some STIs are known to be asymptomatic (no symptoms). An asymptomatic person is still able to transmit an STI to others.

I am going to be honest; if it were not for me authoring this book, I would not know any of these statistics. I would have never read any articles on STIs with emphasis on the black population. In fact, I am unsure if a lot of people look up facts on black people and STIs randomly. This chapter was not originally in the plan for this book; however, this is particularly important, and people need to understand the importance of protecting themselves from STIs.

Overall, we must ensure that our people are educated and aware of the risks and the possibilities when engaging in any type of sexual relationship. It is important that you always know your STI status. If you need to be tested or if you think that you were exposed to an STI or have a symptom of an STI, find a local clinic or contact your physician to get tested and treated right away.

Chapter References

1. Health Disparities in HIV, Viral Hepatitis, STDs, and TB. (n.d.). *Centers for Disease Control and Prevention*. https://www.cdc.gov/nchhstp/healthdisparities/afri canamericans.html
2. Ojikutu BO, Mayer K. HIV Prevention Among Black Women in the US—Time for Multimodal Integrated Strategies. *JAMA Netw Open*. 2021;4(4):e215356. Doi:10.1001/jamanetworkopen.2021.5356

Chapter 29.
Blacks + Incarceration

Did you know that over seventy percent of prison inmates read at a fourth-grade level or less? Are you aware that the fastest growing prison population in the US is women? Although we are only around thirteen percent of the national population, we (black people) make up forty percent of federal prisoners.

For over twenty years I watched my own father, Ralph Cunningham, counsel both men and women straight out of prison. This was a passion for him as he was once an inmate in Jackson State Penitentiary. He worked non-stop to keep individuals from returning to prison. Many of them had struggles with drug and alcohol addiction and this often fueled criminal behavior and created a vicious cycle. Although he could not reach everyone, his results were so unusual that it garnered a lot of attention from those working in law enforcement and in the judicial system. Many asked him what he was doing to help these people change. He had a very specific methodology that he used to help these men and women work to regain their lives.

My father was aware of the system on both sides since he was a former inmate. He knew the mindset and the barriers that many would face. Depending on the nature of their criminal record, many times housing was one of the first issues. He also knew about the barriers to finding employment and was able to help people find work, even those that had been incarcerated for thirty years or longer.

Incarceration has caused many of our children to grow up without the day-to-day love, support, and guidance of their mother and father. Some parents are incarcerated so long that before they can warn their kids to stay on the straight and narrow, they end up incarcerated together - both parent and child. Sadly, I have even seen three generations locked up at the same time. The vicious cycle of poverty, broken homes, negative environment, barriers created by systemic racism, and negative cultural influences are wreaking havoc on our youth. The hopelessness that resides in our communities has left many of our people without a way of escape and without a bright future.

The number of children left without parents due to one or both parents being incarcerated is heartbreaking. It is bad enough when children have a father that is absent or incarcerated. But it can be more difficult when the mother is also incarcerated. This has been the cause of many children being left with grandparents or other family members and in other cases becoming wards of the state. Black children are more likely than any other group to have had an incarcerated parent, and it is believed that about one out of nine black children fall into this category.

One hard reality is that often the family members do not realize that the person that went away is not the same person that will return home. Although we have seen the world of entertainment portray prison in a positive light, that is far from the truth. Living in an environment where men and women are raped, prostituted, blackmailed, drugged, bullied, violently attacked, and murdered, it should not be a shock that people are not the same when they leave.

I will never forget the story that my father told me about his best friend. They were incarcerated together and were supposed to be released around the same time but while he was in his cell on the other side of the prison, his friend was stabbed to death. That traumatized my father greatly and he cannot tell that story to this day without tears streaming down his face.

This chapter was included because incarceration is detrimental to the health of those that are behind bars. Incarceration can have a negative impact on a person's health due to inadequate healthcare, subpar dental care, limited mental healthcare services, and eating a poor diet for years at a time.

So many of our people are incarcerated way too young and for way too long. It is a harsh reality that black people are more prone to being over-sentenced than any other group. Being incarcerated can be very traumatic and hard on a person's mental health. I have seen people go into prison with a sound mind and come out with severe mental health issues that they were no longer able to function on their own.

For several years I worked in a substance abuse counseling agency with individuals that were reentering society after incarceration. I noticed that a lot of the males would typically sit with their back to the wall. They were easily triggered, and many had to relearn society's rules versus prison rules. Many expressed issues with heightened anxiety upon release from prison. Simple things like going to a large public store or a mall was overwhelming for a lot of people who were formerly incarcerated. After being in prison for years, they were not used to big crowds of random, free-flowing people. Everyone's experience in prison is different, but I have yet to meet anyone that said that they had an enjoyable time, and that nothing ever went wrong.

Whenever the topic of fair treatment for prisoners and felons comes up, there are always individuals that have a "Who cares?" attitude. However, being incarcerated does not mean that they are no longer human. Also, it does not mean that a person cannot turn their life around. A lot of people are enduring long sentences for non-violent offenses. Furthermore, let us not forget how many black men and women were given extremely harsh sentences that do not match their crime, or those that lost decades of their lives for crimes that they never committed.

Incarceration impacts:

Physical health – poor diet, violent attacks, STDs, extremely poor healthcare, poor maternal care, poor/inadequate dental care

Mental health – stress, traumatic events, untreated/undiagnosed/undertreated mental health disorders, no visits or family/friend communication, isolation, anxiety due to the prison environment, suicidal ideation, suicide attempts

Social health – it separates family members; incarceration can add stress to family members at home, losing touch with loved ones, disconnection from spouse and children

Financial health – A lot of people upon release from prison will try to rebuild their lives with zero dollars. Some have had family members steal their money and destroy their credit while incarcerated. Inmate needs and requests can be a financial burden on family and friends at home.

Incarceration has a complex effect on the health of those that are behind bars. However, it can also impact the health of their loved ones. The distance, stress, financial burden, and other factors can impact an entire family significantly.

I am hopeful that more programs and initiatives will be put in place not only to support at-risk youth and those reentering society but will also provide needed programs to support their families.

Stronger, healthier families and support systems could help reduce the chances for some of our people becoming incarcerated. The role of family in our lives as we develop, and the importance of a stable foundation at home is important. Besides, creating programs that only benefit the individual but do not address the home environment, relationship dynamics, and support system might not be as effective. Overall, we must do our part to keep as many of our people as possible out of prison.

Chapter 30.

Sickle Cell Anemia

Data has shown that sickle cell disproportionately affects black Americans. According to the CDC, sickle cell occurs in almost one in three hundred and sixty-five black births, and about one in thirteen are carriers of the sickle cell trait.[1] The majority of people affected by SCD in United States are black people, and being black increases your risk for this disease.

At this point you might be wondering: what is sickle cell disease (SCD)? SCD is a group of blood disorders that are inherited genetically from both parents and is present when a baby is born (it is congenital). SCD is normally diagnosed at birth due to tests and screenings that are conducted on newborns. Although SCD is diagnosed right away, symptoms typically do not begin until babies are closer to 6 months of age. SCD does not affect everyone the same way because complications, symptoms and severity of this disease can vary from one person to the next.

When someone has sickle cell disease, this means that they have inherited **two** sickle cell genes (one comes from each parent). However, individuals with the sickle cell trait (SCT) inherit **one** sickle cell gene from one parent and one normal gene from the other parent. In most cases individuals that have SCT are completely asymptomatic, but they are still able to pass this one sickle cell gene down to their children.

When an individual has SCD and has inherited two sickle cell genes (one from each parent), these genes will code for an abnormal form of hemoglobin that will cause the red blood cells to be sticky, inflexible and sickle shaped. Hemoglobin is a protein that can be found in red blood cells; it contains iron and has an important function to help transport oxygen from your lungs to the rest of your body.

Sickle Cell Disease Complications

When a person does not have sickled cells, their red blood cells will be round, flexible and have no issues moving through tiny blood vessels. On the other hand, a person that has sickle cell disease has sickle-shaped (or crescent-shaped) red blood cells, and when they try and pass through small blood vessels, they can get stuck, and this can lead to a pain crisis (vaso-occlusive episode). These episodes can last for hours, or days, and in severe cases they can lead to hospitalization.

Sickle cell disease can also cause anemia because these cells are known to be fragile (break apart) with short lifespans. On average, red blood cells live approximately one hundred and twenty days, but sickle cells live on average between ten and twenty days. This can lead to a shortage of red blood or anemia which means the tissues in their bodies are not getting enough oxygen.

Other Sickle Cell Complications

- Infections - i.e., Pneumonia, and meningitis. The susceptibility to infections is believed to be associated with spleen dysfunction. SCD can block the blood vessels in the spleen and cause damage. The spleen helps the body fight infections, and it also filters the blood by removing things such as old/damaged blood cells.[2]

- Issues with Vision - small blood vessels that supply blood to the eye can become blocked by sickled cells and cause damage.

- Strokes - Sickle cells can clump together and block blood vessels. This can result in the formation of blood clots, or blockage of major blood vessels in the brain. Blockage to blood flow and oxygen to the brain can result in a stroke and damage to the brain.[3]

- Priapism - This occurs in males and is the result of sickle cells blocking blood vessels in the penis causing an erection. While this is happening, the tissues of the penis are not getting oxygen due to the obstructed blood vessels. If priapism lasts too long (more than four hours) or is left untreated, this could lead to erectile dysfunction.

Other complications include sickle cell nephropathy or kidney injury caused by SCD, leg ulcers, splenetic sequestration, acute chest syndrome, damage to organs and nerves, and lower life expectancy than those without SCD.

Symptoms of SCD

- Fatigue
- Dizziness
- Headaches
- Jaundice
- Swelling in the hands and feet

Treatment

Currently, blood and bone marrow transplants (hematopoietic stem cell transplants) are named as the only cure that can help some individuals that have severe SCD. This cure can come with its own set of risks and is the reason why this option is only available to those with severe complications.[4] Other medications and blood transfusions are also available for those with SCD.

I wrote this chapter because unlike a lot of diseases that I have mentioned, a person cannot prevent SCD because it is fully genetic, and they will have it their entire life. Furthermore, this disease is most prevalent in black descendants of Africa.

Lastly, with this chapter I omitted a lot of things intentionally about SCD such as the several types of SCD (i.e., Hemoglobin SS (HbSS), Hemoglobin SC (HbSC) etc.) to keep it simple and easier to follow. I just wanted to share some understandable facts without diving too deep into this topic.

Chapter References

1. Mayo Foundation for Medical Education and Research. (2022, March 9). *Sickle cell anemia*. Mayo Clinic. Retrieved from https://www.mayoclinic.org/diseases-conditions/sickle-cell-anemia/symptoms-causes/syc-20355876#:~:text=Periodic%20episodes%20of%20extreme%20pain,hours%20to%20a%20few%20days

2. NHS. (n.d.). NHS choices. Retrieved February 26, 2023, from https://www.nhs.uk/conditions/spleen-problems-and-spleen-removal/#:~:text=The%20spleen%20is%20a%20fist,many%20of%20the%20spleen's%20functions.

3. *Sickle cell disease*. Stroke Association. (2022, May 13). Retrieved from https://www.stroke.org.uk/what-is-stroke/are-you-at-risk-of-stroke/sickle-cell-

disease#:~:text=Sickled%20cells%20tend%20to%20stick,the%20bra
in%20caused%20by%20SCD.

4. Ashorobi D, Bhatt R. Bone Marrow Transplantation In Sickle Cell
Disease. [Updated 2022 Jul 11]. In: StatPearls [Internet]. Treasure
Island (FL): StatPearls Publishing; 2022 Jan-Available from:
https://www.ncbi.nlm.nih.gov/books/NBK538515/

Chapter 31.

Breaking Generational Cycles

After hundreds of years of abuse, oppression and nonstop targeting, a lot of black people are recognizing the need for change. Although we have always had our teachers, leaders, intellectuals, and social activists, many are still unable to see the big picture. The big picture includes the acknowledgement of how our past has shaped our present and future. Also, it means swallowing the bitterest of pills that many of our people are still stuck mentally, financially, and geographically.

I do believe that we are at a point where many are beginning to wake up. When using the term wake up, I mean that they are becoming aware. Many black people are becoming aware of how a lot of things that were accepted or considered normal are problematic and harmful to us as a people.

I know that many might disagree, but the black community is a constant target for music, movies, TV shows and entertainment that promotes violence, excessive sex, self-destruction, and chaos. One day I had to realize for myself that no other demographic is given this steady diet in entertainment aside from the black community. Over time, we have come to accept this and see it as normal. In fact, mentioning this will probably get some pushback. However, based on the current state of our families, children, and community, these cycles cannot be ignored any longer. It is time to break the generational cycles. These cycles can be seen in our individual homes as well as within our communities.

Breaking cycles can mean unlearning things that caused you trauma during your childhood, or dismissing bad advice that has been passed down from one generation to another. It can also mean being the first to do something in your family, such as graduating from high school, starting a business, or even moving to a different neighborhood.

So many generations of our people have had to figure things out by trial and error. Now, compare this to other communities that have specific heirlooms, money, property, traditions, values, expectations, and other things that they pass down to their children to keep their families strong, create and preserve wealth, increase, or maintain their social status and teach the same to the next generations.

As a people, many of us are trying to find our way by learning and unlearning. We are evolving and maturing in every way possible so that we can make things better for the generations that will come behind us. Many are toiling and trying their hardest to keep going, and they are pushing to "get up out of the mud." A lot of black adults can attest to understanding as a people where we were, where we are, and that we need to pivot to get to where we should be.

The Next Generation

One way to break cycles is through our children. We have the unique opportunity for eighteen years to mold young minds in a positive way. The best way to break cycles with our children is to teach them everything that we did not know nor did the generations before us. We have a duty to prepare the next generation to navigate society. We should endeavor to do this by giving them a leg up in every way possible. Some people are adamant that the plan is when they turn eighteen, they need to get out. If so, then a financial plan and other things should be in place to ensure that they are able to have at least a fighting chance. Years ago, you could graduate from high school and get a job. However, putting kids out at eighteen with no money saved up, no plan, and no support or real guidance can be a disaster in this fast-paced society that is transforming quickly.

With technology and information all around us, we are in a position where we can learn and make moves for the betterment of our children and families. This could mean tackling poverty mindsets early and false beliefs that keep our people behind mentally and crippled by poverty. It could also mean purchasing life insurance, setting up a trust, saving money, or helping the youth start profitable businesses. My daughter started her first business at the age of fourteen and she is still going. My son is on the verge of stepping into the world of business, and he will be twelve this year (2023). If they are passionate, we must invest and push them and steer them in the direction needed to build generational wealth and break the chains of generational poverty. Our youth are brilliant, and they are as capable as anyone else. Many times, they just need that support, guidance and help to find their path so they can go further than the generations before them.

Family

There are so many cycles that we need to break, and they are not just related to poverty and money. We can break cycles by making better decisions and by addressing issues. The statement, "What happens in this house, stays in this house," has destroyed so many black lives and that is a conversation within itself. These words have allowed families to shame victims while protecting the family predators. I can understand that families need basic privacy, but that saying has crippled and crushed so many of our people because it was a code of silence that protected the wicked and hurt the victims.

Sadly, some of these victims felt afraid or guilty for wanting to go to professional therapy to get help from the trauma caused by family secrets. This is why I have told people for quite some time - do not judge these young ladies when they say they do not know the father of their children. Some are victims that were impregnated by momma's boyfriend, daddy, uncle, brother, granddaddy, or some other man that needs to be locked away behind bars.

Breaking cycles in your family can mean putting boundaries in place when handling toxic people; this includes family members. I have lost count of the number of people that let known rapists and pedophiles have access to their children because they are "family." The mindset of trying to be one big happy family while giving a monster access to children is a significant issue. Sweeping things under the rug and pretending that everything is okay is not a good thing. I have seen so many people ostracized by their family for breaking the code of silence and telling the truth. No family is perfect, but some things cannot be overlooked.

Breaking cycles can also mean getting away from family recipes (foods) and lifestyle choices that have every generation overweight and battling a plethora of health issues. When our eyes are open and when we know better, we must then do better.

If you are (or were) a victim of any form of abuse, please find a mental health professional that specializes in trauma so that you can get on the road to healing. You survived, but now it is time for you to heal and thrive.

Finances

The way that we handle finances can be another cycle that needs to be broken. If how you grew up left everyone in poverty, then it might be time to make some changes. Take a financial literacy class, create a budget, or find some legitimate resources that can help you break the cycle. Your local credit union usually has a lot of resources that can help you get some financial peace. I used to think that things like that were boring and unnecessary. My husband had always talked about finances, and I was like, no thanks. But eventually I got a little older and wiser and I realized that I needed a real plan because I did not want to be working at ninety-nine years old.

One significant financial issue that plagues some of us are shady predatory payday loans and other greedy lending options that take advantage of people. They will charge a sky-high interest rate that can cause people to stay in a vicious cycle. If you do not understand interest rates and how they affect what you pay back over time, then it may not seem important at that moment because you are getting access to some quick cash. Sadly, the interest rate will have you paying back so much more than what you originally received. We must educate the next generation about financial literacy, so that they do not get caught into the web of predatory lending.

You Are The One

ENOUGH already! Every family needs one person who gets to that point and says it stops with me - that one person who is brave enough to go against the grain and try to do what has never been done before in their family. Breaking cycles can be extremely uncomfortable, and family members might ostracize you or say that you think that you are better than them. You are just trying to do better, to find a better path for a brighter future. Every generation should not be left in the same position fighting the same battles blindly and losing. You may have to stop listening to what family and friends are saying so that you can be focused and overcome those cycles one by one. We must realize that people cannot help you get to a place that they have never been.

Learning and growing is necessary to break cycles, so invest in yourself. Therapy is always a way to help you manage unresolved issues or your mindset so that you can spread your wings and soar. Finding a mentor, a coach or someone that can help you move forward in life can also be helpful. Finding like-minded people to be on the journey with you to encourage you is important too. If you are trying to launch a business, get around some trustworthy business-minded people that can support you and help you along the way. For any positive changes that you are trying to make along the way, find some like-minded people with whom you can connect, fellowship, and grow together.

Breaking cycles means going on a new and unfamiliar path so that you are paving the way for those that will come behind you. It is unfamiliar territory, but someone must be the ONE - so why not you?

Chapter 32.
The Power of Forgiveness

Forgiveness: The act of releasing the offense (situation) and the offender (person(s) involved). This includes letting go of all anger and negative feelings towards yourself and others.

What does the research show about the impacts of unforgiveness on your health and mental health? There are several research studies that strongly suggest that forgiveness helps to reduce the risk of heart attack; improves cholesterol levels and sleep quality; promotes a reduction in pain, improves blood pressure, and reduces levels of anxiety, depression, and stress.[1]

The conversation around forgiveness is not always an easy one. Many have been scarred and wounded deeply due to the words and actions of others. When we are hurt, many times we are angry and filled with negative energy towards the individuals that have caused us much harm. We may punish or curse them in our minds, or in some instances, we may make life harder for them such as disallowing visits with shared children, unnecessary court battles, damaging property, or physical violence.

Forgiveness is not easy, but it is necessary because holding negative energy inside can cause harm to your physical and mental health, and it is not affecting the person who made you angry. I have seen people angry for decades and as their physical and mental health declined quickly, the person that they were mad at was out living their best life, unbothered. Forgiving others can be extremely difficult and I have seen some people hold on to the same anger and resentment even after the individual has passed away.

Staying upset and angry keeps you chained to the past mentally. No one and nothing are worth staying angry to the point that it can affect your health and your peace. When discussing the topic of forgiveness there are so many things to consider.

1. Forgiveness does not mean that the individual(s) that hurt you were not wrong or that they did not cause you harm.

2. Forgiveness does not let them off the hook, especially when it is necessary to press charges (i.e., physical violence, rape, thievery, identity theft, and other criminal offenses).

3. Forgiveness does not imply that a relationship will be restored automatically or that trust is re-established.

4. Forgiveness is for you and not for the other person. It allows you to free yourself. You might not ever talk to or see the person again, but you set yourself free when you forgive.

5. Forgiveness can require the introduction of boundaries to avoid being hurt the same way again whether by the same individual(s) or by others.

6. Forgiveness can require you to stand up for yourself for the first time. This is especially important for individuals that have been silenced and bullied by family members.

7. Depending on the nature of the situation, some relationships might not be able to be restored. You might deem it in your best interest to handle some people from a distance.

8. Consider that you want others to forgive you for your wrongdoings as well. We all tend to give ourselves a pass because "that" was not our intention, or we did not mean it like "that." As humans we are prone to maximizing what others have done to us while minimizing what we have done to others.

9. Sometimes you must remember to forgive you. We all make mistakes on this journey that we call life, and we must remember to forgive and love ourselves. We should extend the same grace to ourselves that we give to others.

Lastly, remember that forgiveness can be very hard and that it will take time, as it is a process. It is not only saying, "I forgive," although that is a start. When you have spent years or decades dealing with anger and resentment, it will take time and professional help to assist you in releasing the offense and the offender. I always say that if you hear their name or see them, and those same negative thoughts and feelings rise, then you know that you have not forgiven them completely. But when you can see them or hear their name and not get angry immediately, then you are in a place where you have begun to release all that negative energy out of your life.

Chapter References

1. Mayo Foundation for Medical Education and Research. (2022, November 22). *Why is it so easy to hold a grudge?*. Mayo Clinic.

https://www.mayoclinic.org/healthy-lifestyle/adult-health/in-depth/forgiveness/art-20047692

Closing Remarks

I rejoiced when I got to this page. This book has been a labor of love, and it has been a challenge for me in a lot of ways. The first challenge was my skepticism about some of the research issued about black people in general. Whenever I look at a study about black people, my first question is, how did they determine who was black for their study? Was it self-disclosure, or did they look at their outward appearance and classified them as black? Are they black and from America, or from another country? That can matter because black people from different countries have different diets, cultures, and practices than those of us born into families that have been in America since slavery.

My next pattern of thought is - who conducted the research, what kind of study was conducted, and if applicable, how many participants were involved? Why, because the accuracy and relevance of every article or study about black people can be lacking sometimes. Therefore, I tried hard to get facts and information that were from "credible" sources and relevant.

One thing I discovered is that sometimes-black people can be intimidated or apprehensive to ask questions concerning their health during an appointment or when being seen by a physician or other care providers. Also, I found that a lot of people did not know that they could get a second opinion from another professional and that they have the right to switch to a different provider. So many people feel ignored, overlooked, and unheard, which explains some of the attitudes and the disconnect that many black Americans experience with their healthcare providers.

My number one objective with this book was to pull many of the relevant holistic health facts concerning black people together in one place. Also, I wanted to break down or remove a lot of the jargon and terminology that could be intimidating and hard to digest for some readers.

It is my deepest hope that we will begin to consider the state of our health as a people group and as individuals, and that we will be inspired to make the necessary changes to safeguard our health to the best of our abilities.

I hope that we begin to educate our children so that we can break generational cycles of disease, poverty, and trauma so that we can be holistically healthy in our body, soul, and spirit.

As a people we are strong, we are wise, and we are powerful. May my people soar!

BLACK HOLISTIC HEALTH TIPS

Appendix i

---

1. Get interested in your own health
2. Ask your doctor questions
3. Find a primary care physician that is a good fit for you and try to visit the doctor on a regular basis
4. Prioritize self-care
5. Exercise
6. Work on eating healthier. Talking to a nutritionist and dietitian is great, but some changes can be made on your own.
   a. Consume less sugar
   b. Eat more fruits and vegetables
   c. Drink plenty of water
   d. Do not consume large amounts of alcohol
7. Find ways to eliminate/reduce stress
8. Ensure that you are getting an adequate amount of sleep

BLACK HOLISTIC HEALTH GOALS

PHYSICAL HEALTH:

_____

_____

_____

_____

MENTAL HEALTH:

_____

_____

_____

_____

SPIRITUAL HEALTH:

_____

_____

_____

_____

FINANCIAL HEALTH:

_____

_____

_____

SOCIAL HEALTH:

_____
_____
_____
_____

ENVIRONMENTAL HEALTH:

_____
_____
_____
_____

SEXUAL HEALTH:

_____
_____
_____
_____

NOTES

NOTES

NOTES

NOTES

NOTES

_____
_____
_____
_____
_____
_____
_____
_____
_____
_____
_____
_____
_____
_____
_____
_____
_____
_____
_____
_____
_____
_____

NOTES

www.ingramcontent.com/pod-product-compliance
Lightning Source LLC
Chambersburg PA
CBHW062129020426
42335CB00013B/1158